Focus on Emerging Food Borne Infection

FOCUS ON EMERGING FOOD BORNE INFECTION

VIROJ WIWANITKIT

Nova Science Publishers, Inc.
New York

For permission to use material from this book please contact us:
Telephone 631-231-7269; Fax 631-231-8175
Web Site: http://www.novapublishers.com

Library of Congress Cataloging-in-Publication Data

Viroj Wiwanitkit. Focus on emerging food borne infections / Viroj Wiwanitkit. p. ; cm.
Includes bibliographical references and index.
ISBN 978-1-60456-820-2 (hardcover)
1. Foodborne diseases. 2. Emerging infectious diseases. I. Title.
[DNLM: 1. Parasitic Diseases. 2. Communicable Diseases, Emerging. 3. Food Microbiology. 4. Food Parasitology. 5. Gram-Negative Bacterial Infections. 6. Tropical Medicine. WC 695 V819f 2008]
RA601.5.V57 2008
664.001'579--dc22 *2008023746*

Published by Nova Science Publishers, Inc. ✣ New York

Contents

Preface

This book focuses on the "emerging food borne infection", a common health problem in the aspects relating to medicine. This book covers specifically the clinical aspect, scientific laboratory aspect, public health aspect as well as the social science relating to these important tropical diseases. The common tropical diseases, including other disorders, which relate to the food-borne infectious diseases are summarized, presented and discusses. Data is presented from the molecular to the population scales, as well as additional metanalysis for important topics. In addition, the diagnostic guidelines and clinical practice guidelines of the mentioned conditions are presented.

Chapter 1

Introduction to Food Borne Emerging Infectious Diseases

Food-Borne Zoonosis Diseases, an Important Public Health Problem

Infection is still an important problem in the present day. Food-borne disease is an important group of infectious diseases. A food-borne disease is a disease in which the pathogenic organismic microorganism is transmitted via food. The transmission depends upon the attributes and requirements of at least three different living organisms: the pathologic agent, either virus, protozoa, parasitic organism or bacteria; the food, which harbors the pathogenic organism; and the human host (Figure 1.1). Schlundt et al said that diarrheal diseases, almost all of which are caused by food-borne or waterborne microbial pathogenic organisms, are leading causes of disease and mortality in less developed countries, killing an estimated 1.9 million people yearly at the global level [1]. They stated that even in developed countries, it is estimated that up to one third of the population are affected by microbiological food-borne diseases each year [1]. Of several food-borne diseases, food-borne zoonosis diseases are worldwide mentioned. In scenarioes of food-borne zoonosis, the pathologic agents are usually contaminated in foods that are derived from animals [2]. Presently, medical doctors and medical scientists discuss food-borne zoonotic diseases by considering contemporary influences on food no danger and examining pathogenic organisms at the human/animal interface [2].

Schlundt et al noted that the mainity of the pathogenic organisms causing this significant disease burden were considered to be zoonotic and the occurrence of most zoonotic pathogenic organisms tended to pose expanded significantly over recent years [2]. They noted that the factors involved in such expands had not been well studied, but they were mainly agreed to include changes in animal generation systems and in the food generation chain [2]. Specific factors precipitating the emergence of a food-borne zoonosis disease can often be identified.

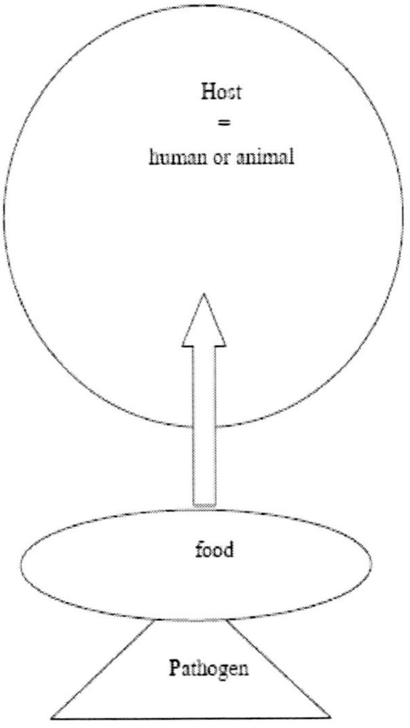

Wiwanitkit, 2005.

Figure 1.1. The composition of a food-borne disease.

These include ecological, environmental or demographic factors that place people in expanded contact with the natural host for a previously unfamiliar zoonotic agent or that promote the spread of the pathogenic organism [3]. These factors are becoming increasingly prevalent, suggesting that infections will continue to emerge and expand [3]. Strategies for dealing with the problem include focusing special attention on situations that enhance disease emergence, especially those in which animals and human beings come into contact, and implementing sucessful disease surveillance and control [3].

Owing to the globalization in the present day, the change in the epidemiology of diseases from one site to the others all around the world can be expected. The summative on the food-borne zoonosis diseases in the tropical countries can be and should be done. That work can be a useful reference material for the practitioners who are not familiar to the unique problems of the developing world and might face up with those problems owing to the possible migration of diseases. Wiwanitkit also noted that the common factor was that all such infections might be transported around the world within their incubation period, and that any disease can now present to any doctor [4]. It is recommended that today, more than ever before, it was incumbent on any practitioner to ask not only "where pose you been?" but also "what did you eat there?" [4].

Table 1.1. Examples of some important food-borne zoonosis diseases

Groups	Examples
Bacterial disease	Salmonellosis, enterohaemorrhagic *Escherichia coli* infection
Viral disease	SARS, ovine spongioform encephalopathy ("mad cow disease")
Parasitic disease	Gnathostomiasis, Opisthorchiasis

Wiwanitkit, 2005.

Owing to the globalization in the present day, the change in the epidemiology of diseases from one site to the others all around the world can be expected. Foods from one side of the world can be easily transported to the other side. The summative on the food borne infections can be and should be done. This work can be a useful reference material for the practitioners who are not familiar to the unique problems of food borne infections and might now be faced with them owing to the possible migration of diseases.

Example of Important Food-Borne Zoonosis Diseases

There are several food-borne zoonosis diseases. The main groups of food-borne zoonosis diseases are bacterial disease, viral disease and parasitic disease (Table 1.1).

Bacterial Disease

In many countries of the world, bacterial food-borne zoonotic infections are the most common cause of human intestinal disease [5]. Thoms said that Salmonella and Campylobacter account for over 90% of all reported scenarioes of bacteria-related food poisoning around the world [5]. Poultry and poultry products pose been incriminated in the mainity of traceable food-borne diseasees caused by these bacteria, although all domestic livestock are reservoirs of infection [5]. White et al noted that the largest number of food-borne disease scenarioes attributed to poultry and poultry products were caused by paratyphoid serotypes of Salmonella and by *Campylobacter jejuni* [6]. The sucessful prevention of these food-borne diseases requires an understanding that contamination can be introduced into foods at numerous points along the food chain [6]. Since multiple entry points exist for food-borne pathogenic organisms, successful control for contamination of poultry requires multifaceted intervention approaches during the various pposeses of the growth period and processing procedure of broiler chickens [6]. White et al noted that it is important to apply risk reduction strategies throughout the food chain and these included: easing the development and implementation of voluntary animal generation "best management practices", implementing in-plant hazard analysis and critical control point systems, developing sucessful transportation and refrigeration standards, and providing educational materials and support for public health activities worldwide [6].

In contrast to the enzootic nature of most Salmonella and Campylobacter infections, *S. Enteritidis* also caused a pandemic in both poultry and human beings during late 20th Century [5]. Holt said that molted hens were 100- to 1,000-fold more susceptible to infection by *S. Enteritidis* and hence more readily transmitted the organism to uninfected hens in neighboring cages [7]. Guard-Petter noted that *S. Enteritidis* is the cause of the food-borne salmonellosis pandemic in human beings, in part because it poses the unique ability to contaminate eggs without causing discernible disease in the birds infected [8]. Guard-Petter mentioned that the infection route to human beings related to colonization, survival and multiplication of the pathogenic organism in the hen house environment, the bird and, finally, the egg [8]. Comparing to *S. Enteritidis*, *S. Typhimurium* and Campylobacter are more ubiquitous in the environment, colonizing a greater variety of hosts and environmental items [5].

Verocytotoxin-producing Escherichia coli O157 (VTEC O157) also emerged as a main food-borne zoonotic pathogenic organism in the 1980s and 1990s [5]. Although infection is relatively rare in human beings, clinical disease is often severe, with a significant fatality rate among the young and elderly [5]. The epidemiology of VTEC O157 is not well understood, although ruminants, especially cattle and sheep, appear to be the main source of infection [5]. Todd and Dundas mentioned that the propensity for VTEC O157 to cause the serious and life-threatening clinical complications of haemolytic uremic syndrome (HUS) and thrombotic thrombocytopenic purpura (TTP), in a significant proportion (2-15%) of affected affected cases, highlights the requirement to focus on it both epidemiologically and clinically [8]. They noted that the fatality rate of these complications (3-17% and up to 30% in outbreaks) added urgency to this concern [9].

The dissemination of *S. Enteritidis* along the food chain is fairly well understood, and control plans pose been developed to target key settings of poultry meat and egg generation [5]. Recent evidence indicated that these control plans were related with an overall reduction of *S. Enteritidis* along the food chain [5]. For VTEC 0157, Hancock et al mentioned that certain farm management practices especially those related to maintenance and multiplication of the agent in feed and water might provide practical means to substantially minimize the prevalence of these agents in cattle on farms and in those arriving at slaughter plants [10]. Unfortunately, existing controls do not appear to decrease the levels of Campylobacter and VTEC O157 infections [5]. Thoms noted that future control strategies required concern on variations in the epidemiology of food-borne zoonotic infections, and applied a quantitative risk analysis approach to ensure that the most cost-sucessful plans were developed [5].

Sorum and L'Abee-Lund said that many zoonotic bacteria carry antibiotic resistance genes directly from different food-producing environments to the human being and these circumstances might pose a main impact on the degree for success in tringesting infectious diseases in man [11]. They noted that several recent examples led to the fact that antibiotics usage in all parts of the food generation chain contributed to the increasing level of antibiotic resistance among the food-borne pathogenic organismic bacteria [11]. They also mentioned that modern industrialized food generation gave addition extra-empposesis on lowering the use of antibiotics in all parts of agriculture, husbandry and fish farming because these food products were distributed to very large numbers of human beings compared to more traditional smaller scale generation [11]. Catry et al noted that antimicrobial resistance might become a main problem in veterinary medicine as a consequence of the intensive use and misuse of antimicrobial drugs [12]. They noted that related problems were arising in human medicine, including the appearance of multi-resistant food-borne pathogenic organisms [12]. They also said that product characteristics, dose, therapy interval and duration of therapy influenced the selection pressure for antimicrobial drug resistance [12]. Basically, there are theoretical, researchal and clinical indications that the new emerged resistance in a pathogenic organismic population can be prevented by minimizing the time that suboptimal drug levels are present in the infected tissue compartment [12]. A series of antibiotic resistance genes pose been sequenced and appeared to be identical or nearly identical in various ecological environments [11]. Similarly, genetic vectors responsible for assembly and mobility of antibiotic resistance genes, including transposons, integrons and R plasmids of similar or identical type are also widely distributed in various niches of the environment [11].

Viral Disease

In 1998, Ferrari and Torres lacking data on food-borne diseases throughout the various countries, with viruses set for being the second most important cause of food-borne diseases in the USA [13] noted that two agents, Norwalk virus and hepatitis A virus, were the fifth and sixth most common causes, respectively. Although the Norwalk virus (NLV) was the sole most common cause of food-borne diseases in 1982 and the second most common cause of water-borne diseases during the period from 1986 to 1988 [13]. Hence, apart from the hepatitis A virus, NLV is becoming more significant [14]. Ferrari and Torres also mentioned that rotavirus, poliovirus, hepatitis E virus, astrovirus, and small gastroenteric viruses are also important causes of food-borne diseases in spite of the scarcity of information on the problem [13]. Because of improved diagnostic means, in particular, and because of molecular biological techniques, viruses can be presently detected much more commonly as pathogenic organisms of food-borne diseases [14]. On an international level means are developed to detect the amount of viruses which minimize polymerase chain reaction (PCR) inhibitors and which are applicable in routine diagnostic usage [14].

Parasitic Disease

There are several food-borne parasitic zoonoses. Both helminth and protozoa infections are mentioned. Sources of food-borne products contaminated with parasitic organisms are pigs, cattle, fish, crabs, crayfish, snails, frogs, snakes and aquatic plants [15 – 18]. The main genera of parasitic organisms are Trichinella, Gnathostoma, Angiostrongylus, Anisakis, Paragonimus, Clonorchis, Opisthorchis, Fasciola, Fasciolopsis, Echinostoma, Taenia, Spirometra and Toxoplasma [15 – 18]. Meat hygienic practice poses become an important instrument of preventive public health since the end of the past two centuries [15]. Parasitic food-borne and water-borne zoonoses contribute to this statistic by inflicting a heavy toll on human health and causing both significant direct and indirect losses to the agricultural industry [16]. The inability of non-industrialized countries to keep pace with population growth, migration from rural to urban settings and the demand for clean, not dangerous drinking water and proper sanitation means that water-borne zoonoses will continue to be an increasing burden of bad health in these developing countries [16]. The consumption of raw or undercooked meat, crustaceans, and fresh-water fish and vegetables can facilitate transmission of large numbers of zoonotic infections [16]. The public health and economic impact of meat- and fish-borne parasitic zoonoses is considerable in terms of morbidity and even fatality in human beings as well as in losses owing to decreased productivity in animals and condemnation of parasitized meat and fish [17]. Cysticercosis, Toxoplasmosis and Sarcocystosis are exposed in detail. With regard to Cysticercosis, the integration of serological means in the inspection procedure could bring a tenfold improvement of diagnostic sensitivity [15]. With regard to Toxoplasmosis, it is obvious that meat containing Toxoplasma-cysts might reach the consumer, as animals infected with *Toxoplasma gondii* can neither be recognized in the ante-mortem inspection nor in the post-mortem meat inspection [15]. About 30-50% of women of child-bearing age are at risk of acquiring the infection during pregnancy with the potential of prenatal infection and severe disease of the fetus [17]. In addition, toxoplasmosis plays an increasing role as an important human immunodeficiency virus-related infection [17]. There are some recent indications that Toxoplasma infections acquired by adults by ingestion of sporulated oocysts might be more pathogenic organismic than cyst-induced infections [17]. Systematical serological investigations on farm level could permit for a proper judgement during meat inspection minimize the consumer exposure to this parasitic organism [15]. Further, reliable means for the detection of Toxoplasma-cysts pose to be developed. With regard to Sarcocystosis, the compulsory inspection of the muscle surfaces to recognize a massive infection with Sarcocystis is still very doubtful in its interpretation [15]. Indeed, there is a need for suitable microscopic, serological and molecular biological means for the detection of Sarcocystis-species and reliable informations on the seroprevalence of Sarcocystis in slaughtering animals [15]. Although cysticercosis is less common the serious presentation as central nervous system infestation is reported [17].

Worldwide, over 50 species of helminthic parasitic organisms from fishes, crabs, crayfishes, snails, and bivalves are known to create human infections [18 - 19]. Eckert said that fish- or crustacean-borne trematodes, especially for Clonorchis, Opisthorchis, Paragonimus and other minute intestinal flukes, infect about 39 million people, and about 550 millions are at risk [17]. Human echinostomiasis, endemic to southeast Asia and the Far East, is a food-borne, intestinal, zoonotic parasitosis attributed to more than 15 species of trematodes transmitted by snails [18]. Two separate life cycles of echinostomes, human and sylvatic, can be demonstrated in endemic settings [18]. The disease occurs focally and the transmission is mainly connected to fresh or brackish water habitats [18]. In addition to echinostomiasis, other serious trematode zoonoses as clonorchiasis, opisthorchiasis, paragonimiasis and fascioliasis are also reported in the tropical countries.

Not only fresh water fish but also marine water fish can harbor the parasitic organisms [19]. Worldwide, the mainity of seafood zoonoses occur along coastal regions where seafood products are commonly ingested [19]. Deardorff said that continuing improvements in transportation, technology, and food handling, however, permited fresh seafood to be shipped worldwide; hence, the high potential for acquisition of parasitic infections from marine products was not limited to coastal populations [19]. Deardorff also noted that the increasing exploitation of the marine environment by human beings, changing dietary habits incorporating natural seafood dishes (including two famous Japanese dishes; sushi and sashimi), and a trend to minimize cooking times when preparing seafood products, could expand the possibilities of becoming infected with these parasitic organisms [19]. Of several marine fish water borne parasitic zoonoses, diphyllobothriasis or fish tape worm infestation is commonly mentioned [20]. The diphyllobothriid tapeworms are primarily restricted to the northern America [20]. Dick et al. mentioned that problems with the specific detection of these parasitic organisms from their fish hosts prompted the development of a series of nucleic acid probes based molecular diagnosis [20].

Tropical Food-Borne Zoonosis Diseases, what and how?

The term "tropical food-borne zoonosis diseases" means those food-borne zoonosis diseases, which are predominant in the tropical region of the world. Indeed, most of food-borne zoonosis diseases are common in the tropical regions. In addition, many common environmental factors in the tropics are related to food-borne zoonosis diseases. Owing to the globalization in the present day, the change in the epidemiology of these food-borne zoonosis diseases from one site to the others all around the world can be expected. The summative on the common food-borne zoonosis problems in the tropical countries is, hence, not limited for the tropical doctors at present.

1. Factor Contributing to the Tropical Food-Borne Zoonosis Diseases

Similar to general disorders in medicine, two main factors contributing to the tropical food-borne zoonoses are inherited and non-inherited factors.

1.1.Inherited Factor

Host Susceptibility

Indeed, the inherited factor poses been widely studied for its role in response to many diseases, especially for the response to tropical infectious diseases. Schlundt et al. noted that the occurrence of some of these zoonotic pathogenic organisms seemed to pose expanded significantly over recent years. [1] They proposed that the factors involved in such expands had not been well studied, but they were generally agreed to include changes in animal generation systems and in the food generation chain and both types of changes could cause corresponding changes in patterns of exposure to the pathogenic organisms and the susceptibility pattern of the human population [2]. In 1991, Del Brutto reported that the main histocompatibility complex played some role in the susceptibility and resistance to parenchymal neurocysticercosis, but the HLA genetic background of affected cases with neurocysticercosis did not seem to influence the severity of inflammatory response against cysticerci, nor was the disease sex related [21].

Susceptibility of Pathogenic organisms

In addition to the host susceptibility to the pathogenic organism, the pathogenic organism susceptibility to the anti-pathogenic organism drug is also widely investigated. For example:

Clostridium perfringens enterotoxin (CPE) poses been shown to be the virulence factor responsible for causing the symptoms of *C. perfringens* type A food poisoning [22]. Genetic studies of CPE pose shown that CPE can be either chromosomal or plasmid-borne and that only a small minority of the global *C. perfringens* population is CPE positive [22].

1.2. Non-Inhertied Factor

Sima Zue *et al.* proposed that in spite of enormous progress in medical science, health care coverage in poor underdeveloped tropical countries remains incomplete, uncertain and minimal and the probability of mortality is high in these countries [23].

In addition, owing to difficult field conditions and limited medical facilities in the tropical countries, proper medical care is often delayed [23]. As the results, most affected cases are admitted with advanced, complicated and untreatable disease to facilities that are often poorly equipped, undersupplied lacking in qualified personnel, and basic medication [23]. These situation also the main problematic concerns for tropical food-borne borne diseases as well.

Poverty

In other words, the poverty leads to lack of opportunity to get good health and bring many health disorders especially tropical infections including tropical food-borne zoonosis diseases. In many developing countries, lack of proper slaughtering facilities and unsatisfactory slaughtering techniques are causing unneeded losses of meat as well as invaluable by-products from animal carcasses [24]. In addition, in many developing countries, regulations concerning meat inspection and control are inadequate or non-existent, permiting consumers to take risk for exposure to pathogenic organisms including zoonotic parasitic organisms [24]. Hence, complex socio-economic and socio-cultural factors significantly impact the maintenance of parasitic zoonoses [25]. Finally, Bhatia said that several factors, including unhygienic living conditions, lack of education, poor personal hygienic practice, poverty and occupation, could contribute to the dissemination of many parasitic infections [25].

Poor Hygienic practice

As already mentioned poor hygienic practice can come from poverty. The population, especially the underprivileged group, in the tropics, usually poses poor hygienic behaviors. Mata proposed that the physical environment in the tropics and the socioeconomic characteristics of the population inhabiting such regions, favor maintenance and transmission of a variety of viruses, bacteria, and parasitic organisms that make agricultural progress and social development difficult [26]. Goh proposed that control of diarrheal diseases was directed mainly at food control and legislation and health education, backed by a high standard of environmental sanitation and a well-set system of epidemiological surveillance [27].

Environmental Temperature and Humidity

Similar to other tropical diseases, the environmental temperature, that is usually hot in the tropics, helps transmit many tropical infectious diseases. Recently, Wiwanitkit done a retrospective study on 33 previous cross-sectional surveys with geographical data and the prevalence of Gnathostoma spp. L3 that covered 12 provinces in Thailand [28]. In this study, the relation between rainfall (derived from the geographical data) and the prevalence of Gnathostomo spp. L3 in swamp eels (derived from the overall infection rate of Gnathostoma spp. L3) was investigated [28]. A significant correlation was discerned between rainfall and the prevalence of eel infection but not for the season of the survey [28]. Wiwanitkit proposed that the prevalence of eel infection might depend on rainfall rather than season [28].

Sposesha and Pammenter studied anticysticercus antibody titer levels among pediatric population from different parts of South Africa; the mean antibody titre level in the dry setting with extreme temperature regimes was higher than that in the wet setting [29].

2. Magnitude of Tropical Food-Borne Zoonosis Diseases

Food-borne zoonosis disease is considered to be a common public health problem worldwide. The tropical food-borne zoonosis diseases show similar high prevalence in each tropical region of the world; however, there might be a difference in the types of disorders. Here, the summary of reports concerning the magnitude and patterns of tropical food-borne zoonosis diseases in many tropical regions is presented.

South Asia

Food-borne zoonosis diseases are important public health problems to many countries in South Asia. Throughout India, problems of food-borne parasitic zoonoses differ because of varied food habits [25]. In the South Asia region vast human populations are exposed daily and with considerable intensity to close contact with vast animal populations and their excreta [30]. Among the commonest zoonotic diseases prevalent in member countries are taeniasis, salmonellosis and campylobacteriosis [30]. Joshi noted that a national plan was needed for each country to give priority to controlling these diseases, based on health systems refind or primary health care, with intersectoral and regional cooperation through the South Asian Association for Regional Cooperation under Technical Cooperation among Developing Countries [30].

Southeast Asia

Similar to South Asia, there are many food-borne zoonoses in Southeast Asia. However, there is a considerable discrimination among the members of Southeast Asia. In Singapore, parasitic infections adopt a rather low profile in the highly urbanized setting [31]. Very few food-borne parasitic infections are encountered. Apart from a few reports of infections with

Clonorchis/Opisthorchis, *Taenia* spp. and hydatid disease, there are no other citations of such helminthic infections [31]. Whereas a number of food-borne parasitic zoonoses pose been recorded in the Philippines including echinostomiasis, artyfechinostomosis, fascioliasis, heterophydiasis, carneophallosis, clonorchiasis, paragonimiasis, taeniasis, echinococcosis /hydatidosis, diphyllobothriosis/spirometrosis and sparganosis, intestinal capillariasis, gnathostomiasis, angiostrongylosis, toxoplasmosis and sarcosporidiosis [32]. Eduardo noted that many tropical infections were endemic in certain settings of the Philippines because of the habit of consuming raw or partly cooked fish, snails, crustaceans, and meat [32]. However, some are now rarely observed whereas others continue to be public health problems [32]. Concerning the Mekhong region, Laos, Cambodia and Northeastern of Thailand, the main problem is the fresh water fish-borne zoonosis [33]. Opisthorchiasis, an underlying cause of cholangiocarcinoma, reaches the world highest prevalence at this setting.

Africa

Food-borne zoonosis diseases are important infectious diseases in Africa. Several studies indicate that toxoplasmosis commonly occurs in Africa, but the epidemiological patterns in these countries are far from being complete [34]. In addition, serological investigations pose been carried out with different means and the results are not always comparable [34]. Food habits, existence or absence of domestic and synanthropic felines, and environmental characteristics of dry settings seem to influence the prevalence of infection in man from 15 to more than 60% [34]. There are only a few reports on Sarcocystis infection in man, whereas its existence in domestic and sylvatic animals is well evidenced [34]. Scenarioes of Sarcocystis pose been identified in some instances but infection is probably underdiagnosed in South Africa [35]. Concerning cysticercosis infection in cattle, it is widespread in Africa with a prevalence ranging from 2 to 50% in relation to breeding and human habits [34]. In South Africa, cysticercosis appears to be most prevalent in the Eastern Cape Province, where pigs roam freely and sanitation facilities are inadequate or non-existent [35]. Segments of tapeworms often feature as an ingredient of concoctions prepared by traditional healers and are suspected sources of many of the scenarioes of cysticercosis in South Africa [35]. In Africa, losses of one to two billion dollars per year owing to bovine cysticercosis pose been reported [36].

South America and Latin America

Food-borne zoonosis diseases are important public health problems in South America and Latin America. In Mexico, for example, porcine cysticercosis is responsible for a loss of more than one-half of the national investment in swine generation and for more than 17,000,000 US dollars yearly in hospitalization and therapy costs for human beings with neurocysticercosis [36]. For all of Latin America, porcine cysticercosis accounts for an economic loss of 164,000,000 US dollars [36].

Some Present Concerns on Food-Borne Zoonosis Diseases

1. Food-Borne Zoonosis Disease in Non-Tropical Countries

The existence of food-borne zoonosis diseases in many non-tropical countries is considered an important public heath problem at present. These diseases are considered as an important emerging infectious problem in the Western hemisphere. Although not a main public health problem, food-borne parasitic zoonoses in the United States are the etiological causes of numerous diseases that occur widely in the population [37]. The most common food-borne parasitic diseases in the United States include trichinosis, toxoplasmosis, taeniasis/cysticercosis, diphyllobothriasis, and anisakiasis [37]. The countries of Eastern Europe including Poland, Germany, Czechoslovakia, Hungary, Romania, Bulgaria, and Albania also face up with the emerging food-borne zoonoses [38]. Of interest, the present status of food-borne parasitic zoonoses in West Germany is characterized by a relatively high frequency of toxoplasmosis, sarcocystosis and *Taenia saginata* infections [39]. It poses been estimated that there could be as many as two million scenarioes of food-borne infections yearly in Germany. Among them are salmonellosis, campylobacteriosis, yersiniosis, infections with verotoxin producing *E. coli*, listeriosis and toxoplasmosis [40]. The possible factors contributing to the changing in the epidemiology of tropical food-borne diseases from tropical to non tropical zone include the good transportation system, travelling and tourism, urbanization, mutation of the pathogenic organisms and the changing of environmental temperature.

2. Co-Occurrence of Tropical Food-Borne Zoonosis Diseases

The co-occurrence of tropical food-borne zoonosis diseases can be seen and can bring a difficult – to - treat condition in medicine. A good example is a co-occurrence between several intestinal parasitic infestations.

Social Epidemiology of Food-Borne Diseases

Food-borne diseases are an important group of diseases that are still the main public health problem of the world. Over the past two decades, the epidemiology of food borne diseases poses changed rapidly as a consequence of changes in the social environment and the ability of pathogenic organisms to adapt to new niches [41]. Several factors pose contributed to the changing patterns of food borne diseases, and addressing food borne diseases will require rapid surveillance and sucessful prevention strategies [41]. Understanding the prevalence and costs of these diseases is important to help set priorities to minimize the burden of disease. The data required for controlling and preventing food-borne infectious diseases pose relied so far on surveillance of the main food-borne infections to follow trends over time and detect outbreak [42]. A wider public health refind approach must also be considered, specifically on the social perception of food-borne risks and the cost-sucessfulness analysis of the prevention measures that are taken [42].

Many advisory reports of the Health Councils in the past century pose dealt, directly or indirectly, with food-borne diseases [43]. For food-borne diseases, social epidemiology is a subject in which it poses a strong interest. Therapy and preventive strategies and plans including social dimensions for food-borne disease are also focused at present. Geographic information tools, biosocial science, and international replication are used to move from a simple correlation to useful prediction of diseases [44 – 45]. Progress usually shows interplay between theory, data, and tools [44]. These innovations are gaining power as they cross disciplinary boundaries, helping to attribute causality to observed relationships, to understand their nature, and thereby to improve the accuracy and usefulness of predictions [44]. For an example of a social epidemiology study on food-borne diseases, Guerin et al [46] studied social consequences of non-typhoid Salmonella. In this work, the authors discussed the right of workers, social benefits, as well as financial consequences of the infection [46].

References

[1] Schlundt J, Toyofuku H, Jansen J, Herbst SA. Emerging food-borne zoonoses. *Rev. Sci. Tech.* 2004;23:513-33.

[2] MacKenzie AA, Allard DG, Perez E, Hathaway S. Food systems and the changing patterns of foodborne zoonoses. *Rev. Sci. Tech.* 2004;23:677-84.

[3] Morse SS. Factors and determinants of disease emergence. *Rev. Sci Tech.* 2004 ;23:443-51.

[4] Wiwanitkit V. Amazing Thailand Year 1998-1999 Tourist's health concepts. Chula. *Med. J.* 1998; 42: 975-984.

[5] Thorns CJ. Bacterial food-borne zoonoses. *Rev. Sci. Tech.* 2000;19:226-39.

[6] White PL, Baker AR, James WO. Strategies to control Salmonella and Campylobacter in raw poultry products. *Rev. Sci. Tech.* 1997;16:525-41.

[7] Holt PS. Molting and Salmonella enterica serovar enteritidis infection: the problem and some solutions. *Poult. Sci.* 2003;82:1008-10.

[8] Guard-Petter J. The chicken, the egg and Salmonella enteritidis. *Environ. Microbiol.* 2001;3:421-30.

[9] Todd WT, Dundas S. The management of VTEC O157 infection. *Int. J. Food Microbiol.* 2001;66:103-10.

[10] Hancock D, Besser T, Lejeune J, Davis M, Rice D. The control of VTEC in the animal reservoir. - 2001;66:71-8.

[11] Sorum H, L'Abee-Lund TM. Antibiotic resistance in food-related bacteria--a result of interfering with the global web of bacterial genetics. *Int. J. Food Microbiol.* 2002;78:43-56.

[12] Catry B, Laevens H, Devriese LA, Opsomer G, De Kruif A. Antimicrobial resistance in livestock. *J. Vet Pharmacol. Ther.* 2003;26:81-93.

[13] Ferrari CK, Torres EA. Viral contamination of food products: a poorly understood public health problem. *Rev. Panam Salud. Publica.* 1998;3:359-66.

[14] Schrader C, Reetz J, Suss J. Food-borne human pathogenic organismic viruses and their molecular detection with special concern of noroviruses and hepatitis A virus in mussels. Berl Munch Tierarztl Wochenschr. 2003;116:496-505.
[15] Lhafi KS, Mitzscherling TA, Kuhne M. Parasitic organisms in meat: a challenge for veterinarians in meat hygienic practice. Dtsch Tierarztl Wochenschr. 2004;111:277-81.
[16] Macpherson CN, Gottstein B, Geerts S. Parasitic food-borne and water-borne zoonoses. *Rev. Sci .Tech.* 2000;19:240-58.
[17] Eckert J. Workshop summary: food no danger: meat- and fish-borne zoonoses. *Vet. Parasitol.* 1996;64:143-7.
[18] Anantaphruti MT. Parasitic contaminants in food. *Southeast Asian J. Trop. Med. Public Health.* 2001;32 Suppl 2:218-28.
[19] Deardorff TL. Epidemiology of marine fish-borne parasitic zoonoses. *Southeast Asian J. Trop. Med. Public Health.* 1991;22 Suppl:146-9.
[20] Dick TA, Dixon BR, Choudhury A. Diphyllobothrium, Anisakis and other fish-borne parasitic zoonoses. *Southeast Asian J. Trop. Med. Public Health.* 1991;22 Suppl:150-2.
[21] Del Brutto OH, Granados G, Talamas O, Sotelo J, Gorodezky C. Genetic pattern of the HLA system: HLA A, B, C, DR, and DQ antigens in Mexican affected cases with parenchymal brain cysticercosis. *Hum. Biol.* 1991;63:85-93.
[22] Brynestad S, Granum PE. Clostridium perfringens and foodborne infections. *Int. J. Food Microbiol.* 2002;74:195-202.
[23] Sima Zue A, Chani M, Ngaka Nsafu D, Carpentier JP. Does tropical environment influence morbidity and fatality? Med Trop (Mars). 2002; 62: 256-9
[24] Joshi DD, Maharjan M, Johansen MV, Willingham AL, Sharma M. Improving meat inspection and control in resource-poor communities: the Nepal example. *Acta Trop.* 2003;87:119-27.
[25] Bhatia BB. Current status of food-borne parasitic zoonoses in India. *Southeast Asian J. Trop Med. Public Health.* 1991;22 Suppl:36-41.
[26] Mata LJ. The environment of the malnourished child. Basic Life Sci. 1976; 7: 45-66.
[27] Goh KT. Epidemiology of diarrhoeal diseases in Singapore. *Asian J. Infect. Dis.* 1979;3:47-56.
[28] Wiwanitkit V. A note on the correlation between rainfall and the prevalence of Gnathostoma spp. infective period larvae in swamp eels in Thailand. *Parasitic organism.* 2004 ;11:401-4.
[29] Sposesha W, Pammenter MD. Sero-epidemiological studies of cysticercosis in school pediatric population from two rural settings of Transkei, South Africa. *Ann. Trop. Med. Parasitol.* 1991;85:349-55.
[30] Joshi DD. Organisation of veterinary public health in the south Asia region. *Rev. Sci. Tech.* 1991;10:1101-29.
[31] Current status of food-borne parasitic zoonoses in Singapore. Singh M, Hian YE, Lay-Hoon C. *Southeast Asian J. Trop. Med. Public Health.* 1991;22 Suppl:27-30.
[32] Eduardo SL. Food-borne parasitic zoonoses in the Philippines. *Southeast Asian J. Trop. Med Public Health.* 1991;22 Suppl:16-22.

[33] Giboda M, Ditrich O, Scholz T, Viengsay T, Bouaphanh S. Current status of food-borne parasitic zoonoses in Laos. *Southeast Asian J. Trop. Med. Public Health.* 1991;22 Suppl:56-61.

[34] Pozio E. Current status of food-borne parasitic zoonoses in Mediterranean and African regions. *Southeast Asian J. Trop Med. Public Health.* 1991;22 Suppl:85-7.

[35] Joubert JJ, Evans AC. Current status of food-borne parasitic zoonoses in South Africa and Namibia. *Southeast Asian J. Trop. Med. Public Health.* 1997;28 Suppl 1:7-10.

[36] Murrell KD. Economic losses resulting from food-borne parasitic zoonoses. *Southeast Asian J. Trop. Med. Public Health.* 1991;22 Suppl:377-81.

[37] Schantz PM, McAuley J. Current status of food-borne parasitic zoonoses in the United States. *Southeast Asian J. Trop. Med. Public Health.* 1991 Dec;22 Suppl:65-71.

[38] Cuperlovic K. Current status of food-borne parasitic zoonoses--eastern Europe. *Southeast Asian J. Trop. Med. Public Health.* 1991;22 Suppl:72-7.

[39] Hinz E. Current status of food-borne parasitic zoonoses in West Germany. *Southeast Asian J. Trop. Med. Public Health.* 1991;22 Suppl:78-84.

[40] Grossklaus D. Zoonoses control--new challenges in health prevention of consumers. Berl Munch Tierarztl Wochenschr. 2001;114:420-7.

[41] Altekruse SF, Swerdlow DL, Wells SJ. Factors in the emergence of food borne diseases. *Vet Clin. North Am. Food Anim. Pract.* 1998;14:1-15.

[42] Desenclos JC, Vaillant V, De Valk H. Food-borne infections: do we need further data collection for public health action and refind. Rev Epidemiol Sante Publique. 2002; 50:67-79.

[43] Mcmichael T. Healthy world, healthy people. People Planet. 1997;6:6-9.Obana M. Food-borne botulism. Ryoikibetsu Shokogun Shirizu. 1999;(23 Pt 1):456-9.

[44] 44. Butz WP, Torrey BB. Some frontiers in social science. Science. 2006;312:1898-900.

[45] Miller S, Diamond J. Social sciences: a New World of differences. *Nature.* 2006;441:411-2.

[46] Guerin PJ, Vold L, Aavitsland P. Communicable disease control in a migrant seasonal workers population: A case study in Norway. Euro Surveill 2005;10: 48-50.

Chapter 2

Taeniasis

Introduction to Taeniasis

Taeniasis is a tapeworm (cestode) disease. Basically, taeniasis is acquired by ingesting raw or undercooked meat of infected animals. Beef generally carry *Taenia saginata* whereas pigs carry *T. solium*. Unlike the beef tapeworm (*T. saginata*), the larval period of the pork tapeworm (*T. solium*) can infect the human nervous system, causing neurocysticercosis [1]. This disease is one of the main causes of epileptic seizures in many less developed countries and is also increasingly seen in more developed countries because of immigration from endemic settings [1]. Little information is available on the natural evolution of taeniasis or cysticercosis [1]. Available therapeutic measures include steroids, therapys for symptoms, surgery, and, more controversially, antiparasitic drugs to kill brain parasitic organisms [1]. Efforts to control and eliminate this disease are underway through antiparasitic therapy of endemic populations, development of pig vaccines, and other measures [1].

Epidemiology of Taeniasis

Taeniasis is an important food-borne parasitic zoonosis that is endemic mainly in Asian and South American countries where some people prefer to eat raw beef and pork. Several reports of affected cases with cysticercosis from many countries in Asia including India, China, Indonesia, Thailand, Korea, Taiwan and Nepal are a clear indicator of the wide prevalence of *T. solium* cysticercosis and taeniosis in these and other Asian countries [2]. However, epidemiological data from community based studies are sparse and available only for a few countries in Asia [2]. Seroprevalence studies indicate high rates of exposure to the parasitic organism in several countries (Vietnam, China, Korea and Indonesia) with rates ranging from 0.02 to 12.6% [2]. Rates of taeniasis, as determined by stool examination for ova, pose also been reported to range between 0.1 and 6% in the community in India, Vietnam, China, and Indonesia [2]. An astonishingly high rate of taeniasis of 50% was reported from an setting in Nepal populated by pig rearing farmers [2]. In addition to poor sanitation, unhealthy pig rearing practices, low hygienic standards, unusual customs including consumption of raw pork is an additional factor contributing to the spread of the disease in some communities of Asia [2].

In Southeast Asia, the taeniasis is still an important food-borne zoonosis. In Vietnam, information concerning porcine and bovine cysticercosis is very limited and based mostly on passive surveillance at Hanoi slaughterhouses [3]. Surveys for human taeniasis in central and northern provinces indicate a prevalence of 0.2-7.2% [3]. However, techniques of low sensitivity were used and the results are inconclusive since it is unknown with which species of tapeworm the people were infected [3]. In addition to *T. solium,* which causes human cysticercosis, *T. saginata* and *T. asiatica* are also known to be present in Vietnam [3]. Willingham et al. said that risk factors investigated thus far with regard to transmission of *T. solium* suggested that consumption of raw pork, inadequate or absent meat inspection and control, poor sanitation in some settings, and the use of untreated human waste as fertilizer for crops might play important roles in Vietnam but this remained to be validated [3]. In Indonesia, taeniasis is endemic on the islands of Bali, Irian Jaya and Sumatra [4]. The Balinese eat pork or beef raw in a dish called "lawar" [4]. It presents half raw pork mixed with coconut and vegetables [5]. Natives of Irian Jaya also pose a custom of preparing and consuming raw pork [4]. On Samosir Island in North Sumatra, undercooked pork is consumed in traditional ceremonies [4]. In Bali, the local people defecate into cages, called "teba", of domestic animals [4]. The prevalence of taeniasis in human beings in Bali varied from 0.8% to 23% and most worms recovered from affected cases were *T. saginata* [5]. Although pork was consumed more often than beef, the prevalence of cysticercosis in pigs and cattle was always low [5]. It was noted that whereas cysticercosis in pigs from 1975-1986 varied from 0.02% to 2.63%, it had not been found since 1986 and the prevalence of cysticercosis in cattle from 1977 to 1981 varied from 0.30% to 2.39% [5]. In Irian Jaya, pigs are permited to feed on human feces inside houses at night [4]. The natives of Samosir Island defecate in their gardens and their feces are easily consumed by freely roaming pigs [4]. Since 1972, studies pose been carried out on the epidemiology of taeniasis in North Sumatra [4]. The *Taenia* spp. found on Samosir Island is morphologically identical to *T. saginata* [4]. However, the local people seldom or never consume beef because it is very expensive, whereas pork is commonly consumed [4].

In South Asia, India is also noted as a highly endemic setting for taeniasis. Indeed, throughout India, problems of food-borne parasitic zoonoses differ because of varied food habits [6]. Other factors, however, including unhygienic living conditions, lack of education, poor personal hygienic practice, poverty and occupation are indicated [6]. Taeniasis is an important food – borne zoonosis in India [2]. In 2002, Prasad et al. studied the human and porcine *T.solium* infection in rural north India [7]. In this work, 72 members of a pig farming community and 50 slaughtered pigs in Uttar Pradesh, India, were examined between November 2000 and June 2001 [7]. Concerning the results, 27 of the human cases (38%) had intestinal taeniasis and 7 (9.7%) had reported seizures whereas 13 of the pigs (26%) had cysticercosis [7]. Prasad et al said that such high prevalences indicated the requirement for detailed assessment of the disease burden in this community [7].

Neurocysticercosis is an important public health problem in South-Central America [8]. Intestinal taeniasis is hyperendemic in several South American countries [8]. In comparison, the prevalence of *T. solium* infestation is lower in India [8]. Singh said that the clinical presentations in several American neurocysticercosis series comprised epilepsy, intracranial hypertension and meningeal-racemose cysticercosis, in roughly equal proportions whereas an overwhelming mainity of the Indian cases presented with seizures and the commonest pathological substrate of the disorder in Indian affected cases was the solitary parenchymal degenerating cyst [8].

Singh also noted for the predominance of solitary forms in India, and of multiproblematic lesional forms in South Central America [8]. Singh noted that the magnitude of *T. solium* infestation and the frequency of pork consumption in a given population appeared to influence the quantum of cyst load in affected individuals [8]. An epidemiological inquiry of humancysticercosis owing to *T. solium* was carried out in Lagamar, Minas Gerais State, Brazil, in 1992 [9]. In this study, a survey of 1109 houses with 3344 inhabitants was made and a history on taeniasis in some member of the family was verified in 300 (34.2%) houses [9]. In addition, stool examinations were positive for *Taenia* spp in 24 (1.3%) of samples examined [9]. In 1995, Silveira-Lacerda Ede et al studied Anti-*T. solium* metacestodes antibodies in serum from blood donors from four cities of Triangulo Mineiro setting, Minas Gerais, Brazil [10]. In this work, a serological survey was done to detect IgG antibodies anti-*T. solium* metacestodes in 1133 sera from blood donors coming from four cities of Triangulo Mineiro setting by the indirect fluorescence antibody test (IFAT) and the enzyme connected immunosorbent tool (ELISA) [10]. Concerning the results, specific IgG antibodies were found in 5.6% of the studied population, showing differences in the positive rates according to their origin: Araguari (13.5%), Tupaciguara (5.0%), Monte Alegre de Minas (4.8%) and Uberlandia (4.7%) [10]. Silveira-Lacerda Ede et al said that the results indicated the probable endemicity of cysticercosis in this population [10].

Taeniasis is occasionally reported in non-endemic setting. Hira et al noted that even in countries where pork consumption was proscribed by religious laws, medical doctors should include cysticercosis in their differential diagnosis in affected cases with neurological symptoms or non-CNS problematic lesions, especially in non-endemic countries with a large expatriate population [11]. They also said that in pediatric population, suspected tuberculous problematic lesions on CT should be investigated to rule out cysticerci by a more diligent use of the sensitive and specific EITB tool [11]. They also noted that failure to understand the local epidemiology leads to empirical, inproper and prolonged therapy for chronic disease [11]. In 2005, community based sero-prevalence study of antibodies to *T. solium* Cysticercosis and *T. solium* Taeniasis in 449 cases living in a federally funded, predominantly Hispanic residential community; and in two migrant farm worker camps in rural Ventura County, California, USA was done by DeGiorgio et al [12]. Concerning the results, the sero-prevalence of *T. solium* Cysticercosis was 1.8% and the sero-prevalence of *T. solium* Taeniasis by serum immunoblot was 1.1%. *T. solium* Cysticercosis and *T. solium* Taeniasis antibodies were not detected in pediatric population [12]. The sero-prevalence of *T. solium* Taeniasis was highest in the migrant farm worker community and handwashing frequency was correlated with *T. solium* Taeniasis sero-positivity [12]. According to this study, the sero-prevalence of *T. solium* Cysticercosis and *T. solium* Taeniasis in this population, as detected by serum immunoblot, approximates the prevalence in some endemic settings of Latin America [12]. DeGiorgio et al. noted that most affected cases likely had prior exposure, not active infection and they said that this study set for the first time, the relative sero-prevalence of *T. solium* Cysticercosis and *T. solium* Taeniasis in at-risk populations in the USA [12]. For the traveler, taeniasis is a precaution for travelling in South America [13]. In 1999, Chatel et al reported a neurocysticercosis in an Italian traveler to Latin America [14]. Similar to South America, the precautions should be applied to many countries in Asia [15].

Concerning the environmental effect on the prevalence of Taenia, Ngowi et al found that prevalence of porcine cysticercosis was considerably higher in pigs reared in households lacking latrines than in those reared in households that were using latrines [16]. Considering seasonal effect on taeniasis, this is no study on *T. solium* and *T. saginata*, however, there was a study on *T. taeniaeformis* [17]. In that work, populations of common voles *Microtus arvalis* were studied as hosts of the tapeworm *T. taeniaeformis* during a 14-yr survey and they were monitored in spring, summer, and autumn in a pastoral ecosystem in eastern France [17]. In that study, a total of 7,574 voles were sampled during 2 multiannual population fluctuations and a third fluctuation was sampled during the expand pposese only [17]. Concerning the results, overall prevalence was lowest in summer (0.6%), expanded by 3 times in autumn (1.5%) and a further 5 times in spring (7.8%) [17].

Genetic and Molecular Biology of Taeniasis

The basic knowledge on genetic and molecular biology of taeniasis is widely studied at present. Molecular variation of *T. solium* in the world is mentioned [18 - 19]. According to the study of Okamoto et al in 2001, complete nucleotide sequences of the mitochondrial cytochrome b (Cytb) and cytochrome c oxidase subunit I (CO I) genes from various isolates of *T. solium* were examined [18]. In this work, 11 isolates were analyzed; two isolates from China, 2 isolates from Indonesia, 1 isolate each from India, Thailand, Mexico, Ecuador, Peru, Mozambique and Tanzania [18]. In this work, in both genes, two isolates from Indonesia shared the same sequences [18]. Similarly, the isolate from Mexico shared same sequences with that from Peru, and the isolate from Mozambique shared same sequences with that from Tanzania [18]. In addition, phylogenetic trees inferred from different mitochondrial genes yielded almost the same topology; both the UPGMA and NJ-trees were also very similar [18]. Okamoto et al said that these trees indicated that *T. solium* might be diverged to 2 genetic groups; isolates from Asia form one group and isolates from Africa and Latin America belong to the other [18]. They also mentioned that *T. solium* prevalent in Africa and in Latin America shares the related origin and had recently been introduced to each setting, perhaps with domestic pigs or human [18]. Nakao et al also reported a similar work in 2002 [19]. In that work, genetic polymorphism was determined among 13 isolates of *T. solium* from various regions using PCR-amplified sequences of 2 mitochondrial genes: Cytc oxidase subunit 1 and Cytb [19]. In this work, the 2 phylogenies obtained were similar to each other regardless of the genes examined. The isolates from Asia (China, Thailand, Irian Jaya and India) formed a sole cluster, whereas the isolates from Latin America (Mexico, Peru, Ecuador, Bolivia and Brazil) combined with those from Africa (Tanzania, Mozambique and Cameroon) to form an additional cluster [19]. Nakao et al said that these results and historical data of swine domestication, distributed apperance of pigs and colonization suggest that *T.*

solium had been introduced recently into Latin America and Africa from different regions of Europe during the colonial age, which started 500 years ago, and that the tapeworm of another origin independently spread in Asian countries [19].

For *T. saginata*, Bernitez et al. found that sequence and immunogenicity of the *T. saginata* was homologue of the main surface antigen of *Echinococcus* spp [20].

In this work, a clone (R-Tso18) was isolated from a *T. saginata* oncosphere cDNA library by screening with sera from rabbits immunised with oncosphere extract and it contained a full-length cDNA sequence of 1893 bp with an open reading frame of 1680 bp, corresponding to 559 amino acids with a deduced molecular mass of 65.173 kDa and an isoelectric point of 6.08 [20]. Concerning the results, the R-Tso18 protein showed 80-84% nucleotide identity with the main protoscolex surface antigens of Echinococcus multilocularis (EM10) and E. granulosus (EG10) [20]. In addition, preliminary immunogenicity studies employing the radiolabeled R-Tso18 protein in immune co-precipitation tools indicated sero-positivity for T. saginata-infected calf sera (6/13), T. solium cysticercosis human (7/22) and pig (2/2) sera and E. multilocularis (6/10)- and E. granulosus (1/12)-infected human sera, whereas other helminth-infection sera were negative [20]. Benitez et al concluded that further studies on the diagnostic potential of the purified recombinant R-Tso18 antigen, or its peptides, were merited [20]. In 1990, Harrison et proposed a differential diagnosis of *T. saginata* and *T. solium* with DNA probes [21]. In this work, a size selected genomic DNA library was constructed using DNA extracted from *T. saginata* then the DNA was digested using the restriction enzyme EcoR1 under star conditions and the 2-4 kbase fraction, selected following sucrose density-gradient separation, was cloned in the bacteriophage lambda gt 10 [21]. In this work, a panel of cestode DNAs including *T. saginata*, *T. solium*, *T. taeniaeformis*, *T. crassiceps*, Echinococcus granulosus and DNAs of bovine, porcine and human origin were used in conjunction with hybridization analysis to identify two recombinant bacteriophages [21]. Concerning the results, the first probe, designated HDP1, reacted specifically with *T. saginata* DNA whereas the second, designated HDP2, reacted with DNA from *both T. saginata* and *T. solium* but not the other DNA samples and thus provided a general reagent for positive detection of fragments of *Taenia* spp. proglottides of human faecal origin [21]. Harrison et al. said that it was important to be able to distinguish *T. saginata* and *T. solium* infections in clinical situation and DNA probes including these might be useful in such differentiation [21].

In additional to *T. solium* and *T. saginata*, recent studies on the epidemiologic pattern of taeniasis in Southeast Asia pose indicated the existence of a third form of human Taenia, distinguishable from *T. saginata* and *T. solium* [22]. Originally termed Taiwan Taenia, and first described in Taiwanese aboriginals, this newly recognized taeniid is now generally referred to as Asian Taenia since it poses since been recorded in a number of other Asian countries [22]. In 1994, Bowles and McManus used a genetic yardstick approach to determine whether the Asian Taenia should most properly be considered as a new, distinct species or as a subspecies, strain, or variant of *T. saginata*, which previous studies pose shown it closely resembles [22]. In this work, sequence variation in the 28S rRNA and mitochondrial Cytc oxidase I (COI) genes of a range of taeniid cestodes and the COI and rDNA internal transcribed spacer I PCR restriction fragment length polymorphism (RFLP) pattern differences in the Asian Taenia, T. saginata, and T. solium were used as markers of genetic identity [22]. Concerning the results, the PCR-RFLP approaches proved useful for rapid and unambiguous discrimination of Asian Taenia from the other two human species, whereas the mitochondrial and nuclear sequence comparisons indicate that the Asian Taenia was much more closely related to *T. saginata* than recognized taeniid species were to each other [22]. Bowles and McManus said that the results support earlier conclusions that the Asian Taenia was a genetically distinct entity but is closely related to *T. saginata*, and suggest that its taxonomic classification as a subspecies or strain of *T. saginata* was more proper than formal designation as a new species [22]. They also mentioned that the very close relationship between Asian Taenia and *T. saginata* had public health implications in that the Asian form was unlikely to be an important cause of human cysticercosis because *T. saginata* cysticercosis, if it occurred at all in human beings, was an extremely rare phenomenona [22].

Pathophysiology and Clinical Presentation

1. Basic Knowledge on the Pathogenic organism

Taenia spp is classified in cestode group. Of several species, *T. solium, T. saginata* and *T. asiatica* are the three main problematic parasitic organism to human beings. Concerning *T. saginata*, the adult tapeworms pose an average length of about 5 meters, consisting of approximately 1000 proglottids, but might grow up to 17 metres in length occasionally, and are, hence, longer than the adult forms of *T. solium* [23]. The mature proglottids pose approximately double the number of testes that *T. saginata* poses and are larger [23]. The gravid proglottids are also larger, measuring approximately 20mm long by 6mm wide, pose a uterus with more lateral branches, less than *T. solium* [23]. These gravid proglottids when detached from the strobila might be very active, not only crawling away from the feces when passed, but often actively emerging from the anus to deposit eggs from the ruptured uterus around the perianal region [23]. The scolex in this tapeworm might also be differentiated from *T. solium* as it is slightly larger, at approximately 2mm in diameter, and is unarmed, without any hooks, although the 4 acetabular suckers are still present [23]. Concerning *T. solium*, the adult tapeworms pose an average length of about 3 meters, but might grow up to 8 metres in length occasionally, and follow the typical morphology of cestode tapeworms [23]. The strobila presents between 800 and 1000 proglottids [23]. The mature proglottids having trilobed ovaries with a small central lobe in addition to the two lateral lobes and only approximately half the number of testes that *T. saginata* poses [23]. The gravid proglottids, measuring approximately 12mm long by 6mm wide, pose a uterus with between 8 to 12 lateral branches, less than T. saginata [23]. The scolex in this tapeworm might also be differentiated from *T. saginata* as it is equipped with a low rostellum with a double crown of approximately 30 hooks [23]. Concerning *T. asiatica*, Eom and Rim

Said that *T. asiatica* was different morphologically from *T. saginata* in having the unarmed rostellum on the scolex of adult, the large number of uterine twigs and the existence of posterior protuberance [24]. They noted that these structures in the gravid proglottids were used as taxonomic keys in taeniid tapeworms for the first time [24]. Eom and Rim also said that *T. asiatica* metacestode (*Cysticercus viscerotropica*) was different morphologically from

T. saginata metacestode (*Cysticercus bovis*) in having wartlike formations on the external surface of the bladder wall [24]. In addition, Eom et al demonstrated that T. asiatica was sympatrically distributed with the other 2 species of Taenia in the human host in mainland China [25]. As previously described all of the three *Taenia* spp can cause intestinal taeniasis but only *T. solium* poses the neurological presentation, cysticercosis.

Concerning the life cycle of *T. solium*, pigs raised in unsanitary conditions (access to human feces) might contain cysticerci or bladder worms embedded in their muscles (meat) and when a bladder worm is ingested, the gastric juice of the stomach dissolves the wall of the capsule, releasing the inside scolex [26]. The scolex turns inside out and attaches by suckers and hooks to the wall of the intestine and it then begins to create buds, called proglottids, at its posterior [26]. These remain attached to each other for a time and, as they mature, each develops both male and female sex organs [26]. Although there are rudimentary nervous, excretory, and muscular structures shared by the proglottids, each can be considered a separate sexually-reproducing individual [26]. The most mature proglottids eventually break loose and are passed eggs out in the feces [26]. Fertilized eggs released by the shed proglottids might reach the soil ready to be consumed by a pig [26]. However, if tapeworm eggs should be ingested by a human instead of a pig (not all that rare in regions with poor sanitation), cysticerci can still develop and these might form large cysts - often in the brain, neurocysticercosis, which can be life-threatening [26].

Concerning the life cycle of *T. saginata*, the life cycle is similar to *T. solium* but cattle, instead of pigs, raised in unsanitary conditions accessible to human feces. Also, there is no human to human fecal-oral transmission in *T. saginata*. Concerning *T. asiatica*, man is the only definite host of this parasitic organism and the domestic pig and wild boar in Taiwan as well as the domestic pig in Korea pose been determined to be the natural intermediate hosts [27]. Moreover, the pig poses been demonstrated to be the most favorable researchal intermediate host and the cysticerci are situated mainly in the liver [27].

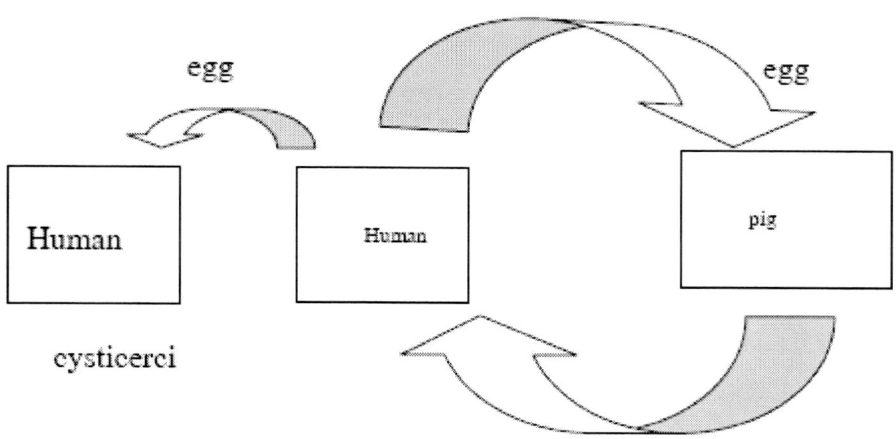

Wiwanitkit V, 2005.

Figure 1. Diagram for life cycle of *T. solium*.

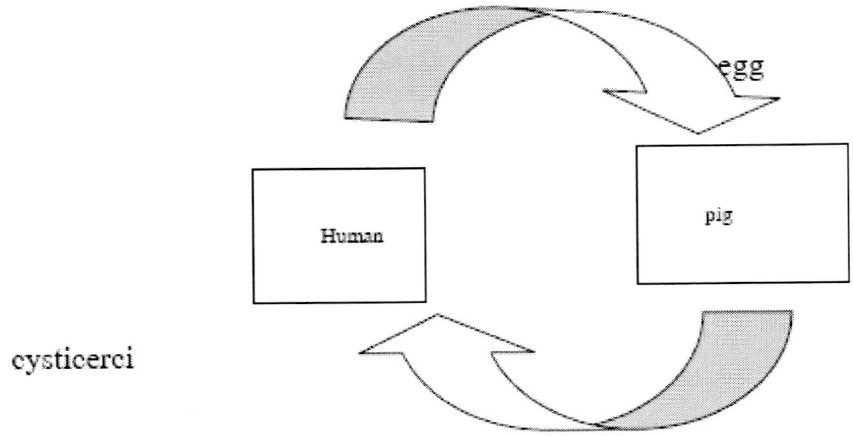

Wiwanitkit V, 2005.

Figure 2. Diagram for life cycle of *T. saginata*.

Considering the cysticerci, they are smaller than *T. saginata* cysticerci and pose a shorter developmental period of four weeks [27]. The scolex of Asian Taenia cysticercus is often armed with two rows of hooklets [27]. The adult worm of Asian Taenia is shorter and poses less number of segments than the classical *T. saginata* [27]. The infection of Asian Taenia can be prevented by avoiding to eat raw or undercooked meat and viscera of pigs in the endemic regions [27].

2. Pathophysiology of Taeniasis

Taeniasis is a parasitic disease that is caused by the ingestion of contaminated raw pork or meat. Avila et al. reported an interesting animal research to study inflammatory responses in the intestinal mucosa of gerbils and hamsters researchally infected with the adult period of *T. solium* [28]. They found that expulsion of *T. solium* in gerbils and hamsters might be related to the expand of goblet cells and mast cells, but these cells might pose different roles in each rodent model of taeniasis [28]. In 2003, Avila et al also done another interesting research to study kinetics of *T. solium* antibodies and antigens in researchal taeniasis [29]. According to this work, they mentioned that the existence of IgG antibodies indicated that tapeworms induced an immune response in the researchal host and that when hamsters were suppressed with corticosteroids the immune response was impaired and did not permit the detection of IgG coproantibodies [29]. They indicated, in addition, that the passage of *T. solium* antigens from the small intestine to the circulation was blocked [29].

Concerning the neurological involvement of *T. solium*, cysticercosis, infection occurs following oral ingestion of eggs of the porcine tapeworm, *T. solium* [30]. Consequently, eggs migrate to distal tissue sites via the bloodstream, and develop into larval cysts [30]. When cyst growth disrupts normal function of the CNS, affected cases most commonly present with new onset seizures or hydrocephalus [30].

3. Clinical Presentation

The main clinical presentation for all taeniasis is the intestinal taeniasis. Considering intestinal taeniasis, most of the scenarioes are asymptomatic. The most common complaint is passage (active or passive) of proglottids, which is related with slight discomfort. Other symptoms include colicky abdominal pain (more common in pediatric population), nausea and diarrhea. For *T. solium*, the neurocysticerosis is another important clinical presentation. Indeed, neurocysticercosis is the commonest parasitic disease of the human nervous system. Immunological tools detect positivity for human cysticercosis in 8-12% of people in some endemic regions, which indicates the existence of antibodies against the parasitic organism but not necessarily active or central-nervous-system infection [31]. The only reliable tool for diagnosis of neurocysticercosis is imaging by CT or MRI. The existence of viable cysts with a mural nodule, related with degenerative cysts and calcifications, is typical [31]. Classification of neurocysticercosis into active, transitional, and inactive forms gives a good clinical-imaging correlation and facilitates medical and surgical therapy [31]. The main clinical presentations of neurocysticercosis are seizures, headache, and focal neurological deficits, and it can pose such sequelae as epilepsy, hydrocephalus, and dementia [31]. Recently, Dhamija et al reported a clinical spectrum of 58 scenarioes of neurocysticercosis in India [32]. In this series, the initial presentation was seizure disorder (33), raised intracranial tension (19), meningoencephalitis (5) and psychiatric presentation (1) [32].

Diagnosis of Taeniasis

For intestinal taeniasis, direct clinical or laboratory evidence of the etiologic agent is usually by microscopic mean. The determination of the *Taenia* spp in the affected case's stool is the clue for diagnosis of intestinal taeniasis. Morphologically, eggs of *Taenia* spp. (saginata and solium) are identical, spherical (30-45 μm), brown to dark-yellow with a thick shell wall and contain an onchosphere [23, 26]. To identify the specific species, the proglottids should be available. For getting proglottids, laxatives should be prescribed for the affected cases the special collection of the stool, and whole stool collection without passing into the toilet, is recommended. The immunological diagnosis becomes the useful alternative diagnostic technique. There pose been a number of advances in immunodiagnosis of taeniasis over recent years that pose improved both diagnostic sensitivity and specificity [33]. Techniques for the detection of *Taenia* specific coproantigens in human taeniasis infections pose been shown to more than double the numbers of T. solium scenarioes accurately diagnosed in epidemiological studies [33]. More recently, work on the serological diagnosis of *T. solium* pose led to the development of a sensitive and specific enzyme connected immuno-transfer blot for the detection of species and period specific circulating antibodies to adult worm excretory-secretory antigens [33]. In addition, "Discharge of proglottids" is the most important clinical presentation, which is also useful in the diagnosis [27].

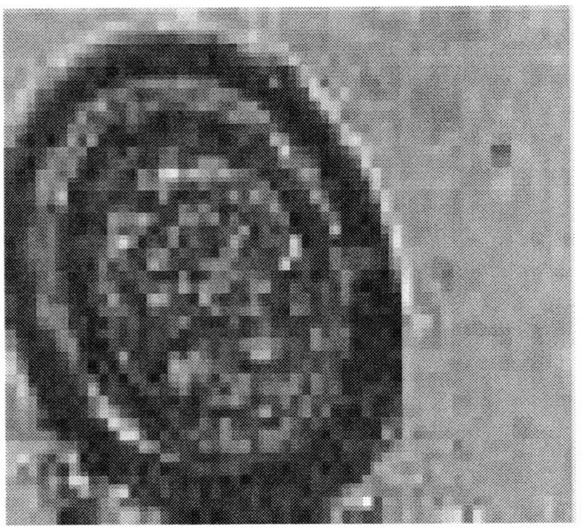

Wiwanitkit V, 2005.

Figure 3. Microscopic view of a Taenia spp egg (x 400).

Concerning neurocysticercosis, a main diagnostic problem with neurocysticercosis is its pleomorphic nature. The diagnosis of human cysticercosis can be made by radiologic imaging, tissue biopsy, or serology [34]. However, radiologic imaging, including MRI and CT, currently is the most sucessful means for diagnosis [30, 34]. Since conventional diagnosis of neurocysticercosis still requires brain-CTand/or MRI, it is often prohibitively expensive and inaccessible in endemic settings. For cysticercosis, immunodiagnostic techniques include detection means for specific antibodies and for circulating parasitic organism antigen in serum or cerebrospinal fluid (CSF) [35]. The antigens used in immunoblot and ELISA for antibody detection pose evolved from crude extracts to highly purified specific fractions and recombinant antigens of the glycoprotein family, increasing both the sensitivity and the specificity of the tests [35]. The application of ELISA for the detection of circulating parasitic organism antigens might present some diagnostic advantages since it demonstrates not only exposure but also active infections [35]. Dorny et al mentioned that only a few of the current techniques had been standardised and fully validated, making comparisons between studies difficult and the lack of a gold standard was a serious drawback [35]. In surveys on cysticercosis, antibody detection systems pose been useful in identifying the risk factors related with transmission of *T. solium*; a high seroprevalence in a community indicates a "hot spot" where preventive and control measures should be applied, in contrast, the potential use of immunodiagnostic tools to identify scenarioes of neurocysticercosis in man is subject to debate [35]. Dorny et al. said that the correlation between a positive serology and neurological symptoms and/or problematic lesions indicative for neurocysticercosis on neuro-imaging techniques was poor to fair in most studies and this might be implyed by the unpredictable clinical outcome of the infection and the variable immunological response of the human host to infection [35]. However, Dorny et al mentioned that a main problem was that in many developing countries, neuro-imaging means are inaccessible and/or too expensive for the rural population at risk hence serology might provide the only tool for diagnosis of the infection under these conditions [35].

Considering the CSF profile in neurocysticercosis, eosinophilia was observed in about 52.9% [36]. Wiwanitkit said that CSF cytology profile is not a useful diagnostic test for neurocysticercosis [37]. In 2003, Fleury et al. noted that the monoclonal antibody HP10 antigen-trapping ELISA, which poses been used successfully to detect viable Taenia solium cysticercosis, was useful in detection of secreted cysticercal antigen in CSF [38].

Concerning the CT and MRI for diagnosis of neurocysticercosis, these techniques demonstrate the number and topography of problematic lesions, their period of involution, and the degree of inflammatory reaction of the host against the parasitic organisms and pose largely replaced previous radiological procedures including plain roentgenograms, pneumoencephalograms, cerebral angiography and myelography [39]. Image findings of neurocysticercosis are various, depending on the location (parenchymal, cisternal, ventricular, and spinal forms), and temporal evolutional periods (vesicular, colloid vesicular, granular nodular, and nodular calcified periods) of the worm [40]. In general, MRI provides better image detection and definition. The possibility of multiplanar reconstruction of images, its capability to visualize the posterior fossa without bone artifacts, and its high contrast resolution (far superior to that of CT) permit MRI to recognize many forms of cysticercosis not visualized on CT [39]. However, the costs of MRI are high and the equipment is scarcely available in many endemic countries, and its sensitivity for the detection of calcified problematic lesions is poor [39]. CT remains the best screening neuroimaging procedure for affected cases with suspected neurocysticercosis, and MRI is the imaging modality of choice for the evaluation of affected cases with intraventricular cysticercosis, brainstem cysts and small cysts located over the convexity of cerebral hemispheres [39]. Its better image definition also suggests that MRI is superior to CT in the follow-up of the affected cases after therapy [39].

In 2001, Del Brutto et al proposed diagnostic criteria for neurocysticercosis based on objective clinical, imaging, immunologic, and epidemiologic data [41]. These include four categories of criteria stratified on the basis of their diagnostic strength, including the following: 1) absolute--histologic demonstration of the parasitic organism from biopsy of a brain or spinal cord problematic lesion, cystic problematic lesions showing the scolex on CT or MRI, and direct visualization of subretinal parasitic organisms by funduscopic examination; 2) main--problematic lesions highly suggestive of neurocysticercosis on neuroimaging studies, positive serum enzyme-connected immunoelectrotransfer blot for the detection of anticysticercal antibodies, resolution of intracranial cystic problematic lesions after therapy with albendazole or praziquantel, and spontaneous resolution of small sole enhancing problematic lesions; 3) minor--problematic lesions compatible with neurocysticercosis on neuroimaging studies, clinical presentations suggestive of neurocysticercosis, positive CSF enzyme-connected immunosorbent tool for detection of anticysticercal antibodies or cysticercal antigens, and cysticercosis outside the CNS; and 4) epidemiologic--evidence of a household contact with *T. solium* infection, individuals coming from or living in an setting where cysticercosis is endemic, and history of common travel to disease-endemic settings [41]. Interpretation of these criteria permits two degrees of diagnostic certainty: 1) definitive diagnosis, in affected cases who pose one absolute criterion or in those who pose two main plus one minor and one epidemiologic criterion; and 2) probable diagnosis, in affected cases who pose one main plus two minor criteria, in those who pose one main plus one minor and one epidemiologic criterion, and in those who pose three minor plus one epidemiologic criterion [41].

Pathology and Complication

Concerning pathology of intestinal taeniasis, the pathology of intestine is usually not severe. However, the severe pathology can be seen in some scenarioes.

Jongwutiwes et al. reported a case of jejunal perforation caused by infection with taeniid tapeworm possessing unusual morphology that poses not been previously described [42]. In this case, among five cestodes recovered during operation, one exhibited a bifurcation at the posterior end and the other harbored a lateral branching of immature segments from the main strobila [42]. By further sequence analysis of the mitochondrial cytochrome c oxidase I gene and the 28S rRNA gene poses confirmed them to be Taenia saginata saginata [42]. Considering the complication of intestinal taeniasis, appendicitis is the most common complication [43 - 44]. In additional to acute appendicitis, Meckel's diverticulitis is also reported as a complication of intestinal taeniasis [45].

Concerning the neurocysticercosis, ischaemic cerebrovascular disease is a relatively common but under-assigned complication of neurocysticercosis [46]. It is usually caused by inflammatory occlusion of the arteries at the base of the brain secondary to cysticercotic arachnoiditis [46]. In most scenarioes, the involved vessels are of small diameter and the neurological picture is limited to a lacunar syndrome secondary to a small cerebral infarct [46]. However, large infarcts related to the occlusion of the middle cerebral artery or even the internal carotid artery pose also been reported in this setting [46]. CT and CSF examination usually support the cause-and-effect relationship between neurocysticercosis and the cerebral infarct by showing abnormalities compatible with cysticercotic arachnoiditis [46]. An accurate diagnosis of this condition is important since early therapy with steroids is advised to ameliorate the subarachnoid inflammatory reaction which might cause recurrent cerebral infarcts [46]. In scenarioes of cysticercosis, seizures occur in persons with only calcified brain problematic lesions [47]. The existence of periproblematic lesional edema poses also been documented in association with calcified problematic lesions in symptomatic affected cases, but the frequency of this complication and characteristics of the affected cases who develop it are not known [47]. Nash et al. found that periproblematic lesional edema was observed in slightly more than one-third of the affected cases, and some affected cases had common, severely disabling occasions and those with an expanded proportion of enhancing calcified problematic lesions were more likely to show periproblematic lesional edema [47]. They proposed that edema around calcified problematic lesions was common in this population and was related with seizures and neurological morbidity [47]. Finally, the worst complication of neurocysticercosis is mortality similar to other neurological parasitic infestation.

Therapy

For intestinal taeniasis, adequate therapy with anthelmintics and general management can result in good outcome. Praziquantel is the drug of choice [27]. Although praziquantel is the therapy of choice for most human trematode and cestode infections, cost factors pose limited its use in developing countries [48].

Concerning neurocysticercosis, therapy regimens are based on cyst location and developmental period, and include supportive care, supportive care combined with pharmacologic therapy, and surgical intervention [30]. Therapy should be individually fitted for each affected case, with antiepileptic drugs, analgesics, corticosteroids, or a combination of these [31]. Anthelmintic drugs (praziquantel and albendazole) are used routinely, but so far no controlled clinical trial poses set specific indications or definitive doses of therapy [31]. Parenchymal forms of neurocysticercosis pose a good prognosis in terms of clinical remission [31]. The most sucessful approach to taeniasis and cysticercosis is prevention, which should be a primary public-health focus for less developed countries [31].

Prevention

Prevention of the taeniasis can be easily done based on the principle of basic food sanitation. The deep-rooted habit as ingestion of raw and poorly uncooked pork and beef should be corrected. Health education is needed. Surveillance of the contamination of the infective period larvae in the pigs and cattle is also important preventive mean. Gonzalez et al. said that interventional trials with massive human cestocidal chemotherapy, therapy of both human and porcine populations with antihelminthic drugs and/or immunotherapy and health education had shown improvements in specific settings but not yet proven to be sustainable in the long-term [49]. In order to ensure sustainability, they noted that any given control strategy towards elimination/eradication of porcine cysticercosis should incorporate economic incentives [49]. Unlike other parasitic infestation, vaccination for the prevention of cysticercosis is proposed [50]. One option to assist with control of the disease is to prevent infection occurring in pigs by vaccination, thereby breaking the parasitic organism's life-cycle and removing the source of infection for human beings [50]. Several approaches are being examined towards development of vaccines against *T. solium*, one of which is the application of recombinant oncosphere antigens [50]. Two different oncosphere antigens, designated TSOL18 and TSOL45, pose been evaluated, each of which poses been shown to induce complete or near complete prevention against researchal challenge infection in separate vaccine trials in pigs [50]. Lightowlers noted that the TSOL18/TSOL45 vaccine had the potential to make a substantial contribution to the control and, potentially, the eradication of human neurocysticercosis [50].

References

[1] Garcia HH, Gonzalez AE, Evans CA, Gilman RH; Cysticercosis Working Group in Peru. Taenia solium cysticercosis. *Lancet.* 2003;362:547-56.

[2] Rajshekhar V, Joshi DD, Doanh NQ, van De N, Xiaonong Z. Taenia solium taeniosis/cysticercosis in Asia: epidemiology, impact and issues. *Acta Trop.* 2003 ;87:53-60.

[3] Willingham AL 3rd, De NV, Doanh NQ, Cong le D, Dung TV, Dorny P, Cam PD, Dalsgaard A. Current status of cysticercosis in Vietnam. *Southeast Asian J. Trop. Med. Public Health.* 2003;34 Suppl 1:35-50.

[4] Depary AA, Kosman ML. Taeniasis in Indonesia with special reference to Samosir Island, north Sumatra. *Southeast Asian J. Trop. Med. Public Health.* 1991 ;22 Suppl:239-41.

[5] Suweta IG. The situation of cysticercosis/taeniasis in animals/man in Bali. *Southeast Asian J. Trop .Med .Public Health.* 1991;22 Suppl:236-8.

[6] Bhatia BB. Current status of food-borne parasitic zoonoses in India. *Southeast Asian J. Trop. Med. Public Health.* 1991;22 Suppl:36-41.

[7] Prasad KN, Chawla S, Jain D, Pandey CM, Pal L, Pradhan S, Gupta RK.Human and porcine Taenia solium infection in rural north India. *Trans R Soc. Trop. Med. Hyg.* 2002;96:515-6.

[8] Singh G. Neurocysticercosos in South-Central America and the Indian subcontinent. A comparative evaluation. *Arq. Neuropsiquiatr.* 1997;55:349-56.

[9] Silva-Vergara ML, Prata A, Vieira Cde O, Castro JH, Micheletti LG, Otano AS, Franquini Junior J. The epidemiological aspects of taeniasis-cysticercosis in an endemic setting of Lagamar, Minas Gerais. *Rev. Soc. Bras. Med. Trop.* 1995;28:345-9.

[10] Silveira-Lacerda Ede P, Machado ER, Arantes SC, Costa-Cruz JM. Anti-Taenia solium metacestodes antibodies in serum from blood donors from four cities of Triangulo Mineiro setting, Minas Gerais, Brazil, 1995. *Rev. Inst. Med. Trop. Sao Paulo.* 2002;44:229-31.

[11] Hira PR, Francis I, Abdella NA, Gupta R, Ai-Ali FM, Grover S, Khalid N, Abdeen S, Iqbal J, Wilson M, Tsang VC. Cysticercosis: imported and autochthonous infections in Kuwait. *Trans R Soc. Trop. Med. Hyg.* 2004;98:233-9.

[12] DeGiorgio C, Pietsch-Escueta S, Tsang V, Corral-Leyva G, Ng L, Medina MT, Astudillo S, Padilla N, Leyva P, Martinez L, Noh J, Levine M, del Villasenor R, Sorvillo F. Sero-prevalence of Taenia solium cysticercosis and Taenia solium taeniasis in California, USA. *: Acta Neurol. Scand.* 2005;111:84-8.

[13] Peate WF, Pust RE. Health precautions for travelers to Mexico. *South Med. J.* 1985 ;78:335-9.

[14] Chatel G, Gulletta M, Scolari C, Bombana E, El-Hamad I, Matteelli A, Carosi G. Neurocysticercosis in an Italian traveler to Latin America. *Am. J. Trop. Med. Hyg.* 1999 ;60:255-6.

[15] Wiwanitkit V. Amazing Thailand Year 1998-1999 Tourist's health concepts. Chula. *Med. J.* 1998; 42: 975-984.

[16] Ngowi HA, Kassuku AA, Maeda GE, Boa ME, Carabin H, Willingham AL 3rd. Risk factors for the prevalence of porcine cysticercosis in Mbulu District, *Tanzania. Vet Parasitol.* 2004;120:275-83.

[17] Fichet-Calvet E, Giraudoux P, Quere JP, Ashford RW, Delattre P. Is the prevalence of Taenia taeniaeformis in Microtus arvalis dependent on population density? *J. Parasitol.* 2003;89:1147-52.

[18] Okamoto M, Nakao M, Sako Y, Ito A. Molecular variation of Taenia solium in the world. *Southeast Asian J. Trop. Med. Public Health.* 2001;32 Suppl 2:90-3.

[19] Nakao M, Okamoto M, Sako Y, Yamasaki H, Nakaya K, Ito A. A phylogenetic hypothesis for the distributed apperance of two genotypes of the pig tapeworm Taenia solium worldwide. *Parasitology.* 2002;124:657-62.

[20] Benitez L, Harrison LJ, Parkhouse RM, Gonzalez LM, Gottstein B, Garate T. Sequence and immunogenicity of the Taenia saginata homologue of the main surface antigen of Echinococcus spp. *Parasitol Res.* 1998;84:426-31.

[21] Harrison LJ, Delgado J, Parkhouse RM. Differential diagnosis of Taenia saginata and Taenia solium with DNA probes. *Parasitology.* 1990;100 Pt 3:459-61.

[22] Bowles J, McManus DP. Genetic characterization of the Asian Taenia, a newly described taeniid cestode of human beings. *Am. J. Trop. Med. Hyg.* 1994;50:33-44.

[23] The pork and beef tapeworms. Available at *http://www. path. cam.ac.uk /~schisto /Tapes/Taenia.html*

[24] Eom KS, Rim HJ. Morphologic descriptions of Taenia asiatica sp. n. Korean J Parasitol. 1993;31:1-6.

[25] Eom KS, Jeon HK, Kong Y, Hwang UW, Yang Y, Li X, Xu L, Feng Z, Pawlowski ZS, Rim HJ. Detection of Taenia asiatica in China: molecular, morphological, and epidemiological analysis of a Luzhai isolate. *Parasitol.* 2002;88:758-64.

[26] Tapeworms. Available on *http://users.rcn.com/jkimball. ma.ultranet /Biology Pages /T/Tapeworms.htm*

[27] Fan PC. Review of taeniasis in Asia. Zhonghua Min Guo Wei Sheng Wu Ji Mian Yi Xue Za Zhi. 1995;28:79-94.

[28] Avila G, Aguilar L, Benitez S, Yepez-Mulia L, Lavenat I, Flisser A. Inflammatory responses in the intestinal mucosa of gerbils and hamsters researchally infected with the adult period of Taenia solium. *Int. J. Parasitol.* 2002;32:1301-8.

[29] Avila G, Benitez M, Aguilar-Vega L, Flisser A. Kinetics of Taenia solium antibodies and antigens in researchal taeniosis. *Parasitol. Res.* 2003;89:284-9.

[30] Bales HW. Neurocysticercosis: migration of a parasitic organism. *J Am Acad Nurse Pract.* 2000;12:240-8

[31] Carpio A. Neurocysticercosis: an update. *Lancet Infect. Dis.* 2002;2:751-62.

[32] Dhamija RM, Venkataraman S, Sanchetee PC, Roy AK, Bhatia HC. Computed tomographic spectrum of neurocysticercosis. J Assoc Medical doctors India. 1990 ;38:566-8.

[33] Allan JC, Wilkins PP, Tsang VC, Craig PS. Immunodiagnostic tools for taeniasis. *Acta Trop.* 2003;87:87-93.

[34] Richards F Jr, Schantz PM. Laboratory diagnosis of cysticercosis. *Clin. Lab. Med.* 1991;11:1011-28.

[35] Dorny P, Brandt J, Zoli A, Geerts S. Immunodiagnostic tools for human and porcine cysticercosis. *Acta Trop.* 2003;87:79-86.

[36] Wang CH, Gao SF, Guo YP. Diagnostic importance of eosinophilia of the cerebrospinal fluid in cerebral cysticercosis. *Chin. Med. J. (Engl).* 1993;106:282-4.

[37] Wiwanitkit V. Cerebrospinal fluid examination and interpretation. *Buddhachinaraj Med. J.* 1999; 17: 42 – 52.

[38] Fleury A, Hernandez M, Fragoso G, Parkhouse RM, Harrison LJ, Sciutto E. Detection of secreted cysticercal antigen: a useful tool in the diagnosis of inflammatory neurocysticercosis. *Trans R Soc. Trop. Med. Hyg.* 2003;97:542-6.

[39] Garcia HH, Del Brutto OH. Imaging findings in neurocysticercosis. *Acta Trop.* 2003;87:71-8.

[40] Chang KH, Han MH. MRI of CNS parasitic diseases. *J. Magn. Reson. Imaging.* 1998;8:297-307.

[41] Del Brutto OH, Rajshekhar V, White AC Jr, Tsang VC, Nash TE, Takayanagui OM, Schantz PM, Evans CA, Flisser A, Correa D, Botero D, Allan JC, Sarti E, Gonzalez AE, Gilman RH, Garcia HH. Proposed diagnostic criteria for neurocysticercosis. *Neurology.* 2001;57:177-83.

[42] Jongwutiwes S, Putaporntip C, Chantachum N, Sampatanukul P. Jejunal perforation caused by morphologically abnormal Taenia saginata saginata infection. *J. Infect.* 2004;49:324-8.

[43] Sartorelli AC, da Silva MG, Rodrigues MA, da Silva RJ. Abstract Appendiceal taeniasis presenting like acute appendicitis. *Parasitol. Res.* 2005;97:171-2.

[44] Panzeri A, Castoldi F, Undiano C. Acute apendicitis owing to taeniasis (Taenia solium). *Med. Panam.* 1965;23:112-3

[45] Chirdan LB, Yusufu LM, Ameh EA, Shehu SM. Meckel's diverticulitis owing to Taenia saginata: case report. *East Afr. Med .J.* 2001;78:107-8.

[46] Del Brutto OH. Cysticercosis and cerebrovascular disease: a review. *J. Neurol. Neurosurg Psychiatry.* 1992;55:252-4.

[47] Nash TE, Pretell J, Garcia HH. Calcified cysticerci provoke periproblematic lesional edema and seizures. *Clin. Infect. Dis.* 2001;33:1649-53.

[48] King CH, Mahmoud AA. Drugs five years later: praziquantel. *Ann. Intern. Med.* 1989;110:290-6.

[49] Gonzalez AE, Garcia HH, Gilman RH, Tsang VC; Cisticercosis Working Group in Peru. Control of Taenia solium. *Acta Trop.* 2003;87:103-9.

[50] Lightowlers MW. Vaccination for the prevention of cysticercosis. *Dev. Biol.* (Basel). 2004;119:361-8.

Chapter 3

Fluke Infestation 1: Liver Fluke

Introduction to Liver Fluke Infestation

Liver fluke infestation is an helminthic zoonotic disease that poses been increasingly reported in travelers returning from the endemic settings. *Opisthorchis viverrini* is the main causative agent of human liver fluke infestation, a parasitic zoonosis with a great variety of clinical presentations [1 – 3]. Generally, human beings are infected by consumption of infective-period larvae (metacercariae) of *O. viverrini* in infected hosts in the form of partially cooked or uncooked food. In general, this infection is found mainly in Southeast Asia where raw and pickled fish are part of the diet [1 - 4]. It is owing to the consumption of raw or insufficiently cooked fish, contaminated with larvae of the *O. viverrini* [1 - 4]. Once confined primarily to Southeast Asia, liver fluke infestation now is a public health concern in other non endemic countries owing to the high rate of migration [5].

Presently, opisthorchiasis is an important intestinal parasitic organism infection with high prevalence in tropical countries, especially Thailand [6]. It might be connected to the very high incident rate of cholangio-carcinoma in the Northeast of Thailand [7]. *Opisthorchis viverrini* is the main causative agent of human opisthorchiasis. The clinical presentations in human opisthorchiasis is not severe. However, its important complication, cholangiocarcinoma, provided severe presentation including severe jaundice and hyperalkalinephosphatasemia [8].

Epidemiology of Liver Fluke Infestation

Liver fluke infestation is an important food-borne parasitic zoonosis that is endemic mainly in Southeast Asian countries where some people prefer to eat raw freshwater fish [1 - 4]. Sithithaworn et al. said that opisthorchiasis was an important food borne trematode because of the sheer numbers of people infected and its serious morbidities including hepatobiliary diseases and cholangiocarcinoma [9]. They noted that although infections were identified throughout Southeast Asia, the epi-center is northeast Thailand, where high prevalence coexists with a high incident rate of cholangiocarcinoma [9]. Indeed, *O. viverrini* poses been found to be the only species of liver fluke in Thailand [10]. In 1980-1981 the prevalence in the north, northeast, centre and south of Thailand was 5.59, 34.60, 6.34, and 0.01%, respectively, with an overall prevalence of 14% or 7 million people [10].

Recently, Sriamporn et al. done an interesting study in Khon Kaen, northeast Thailand, where the high incident rate of cholangiocarcinoma was reported [11]. According to this study, the average crude prevalence of *O. viverrini* infection in the sample cases was 24.5%, ranging from 2.1% to 70.8% in different districts whereas truncated age-standardized incident rate of CHCA at ages >35 years varied threefold between districts, from 93.8 to 317.6 per 100,000 person-years [11]. After adjustment for age group, sex and period of sampling, there was a positive association between prevalence of *O. viverrini* infection and incident rate of cholangiocarcinoma at the population level: however, associations between cholangiocarcinoma and active *O. viverrini* infection in individuals pose become hard to demonstrate, because of sucessful anti- *O. viverrini* therapy [11].

Liver fluke infestation is rarely reported in travelers, although the disease remains a main public health problem in Southeast Asia. Yossepowitch et al said that the infection was increasingly diagnosed in countries where the disease was not endemic, specifically in North America with the growing volume of international travel and population migration [12]. They reported an outbreak of acute opisthorchiasis in a family that was infected in a non-disease-endemic setting after ingesting raw carp illegally imported from a highly disease-endemic setting in Siberia [12]. An important problem in emerging of opisthorchiasis in non-endemic countries is owing to the migration of the workers since the migration of foreign workers from developing regions to developed countries might potentially lead to transmission of intestinal parasitic infections [13]. Saksirisampant et al. done an interesting study in Thai workers seeking overseas employment and found that the commonest parasitic organism among these parasitic organisms was *O. viverrini* (28.9%) [14]. Saksirisampant et al. proposed that screening for the parasitic infections among these workers could help to decrease their rate of rejection by the countries in which overseas employment was sought [14].

Concerning the effect of environment on the liver fluke infestation, the seasonal variation of the metacercaria, the infective period larva, is mentioned [15].

Sithithaworn et al. mentioned that seasonal variation in metacercariae was a common phenomenon in settings with both high and low endemicity of infection [16]. They noted that the metacerarial load in fish was positively related with infection levels among human beings [16]. The also mentioned that fecal contamination of the study reservoirs is greatest during the early parts of the rainy season as a result of run-off drainage and coincides with the rapid expand in snail populations [16]. Waikagul said that the prevalence of *O. viverrini* metacercaria in fish decreased markedly during the last decade owing to the successful of control plan [15].

Genetic and Molecular Biology of Liver Fluke Infestation

There are many interesting studies concerning the liver fluke infestation, especially those related to the development of cholangiocarcinoma, its serious complication. Honjo et al noted that although *O. viverrini* was common in northeast Thailand, but less than 10% of the inhabitants developed cholangiocarcinoma [17]. They also noted that animal researchs suggested that *O. viverrini* infection alone did not cause cholangiocarcinoma, and thus other environmental and genetic factors might play a role in causation [17]. In 2005, Honjo et al conducted a population-based case-control study in which sex, age and place of residence were matched [17]. According to this study, Honjo et al. found that polymorphisms of GSTM1 and GSTT1 alone were not related with risk for cholangiocarcinoma, whereas an elevated level of antibodies against *O. viverrini* was the strongest risk indicator [17]. They proposed that infection with *O. viverrini* correlated strongly with cholangiocarcinoma, susceptibility which might be possibly related with GSTM1 polymorphism and alcohol might affect metabolic pathways of endogenous and exogenous nitrosamines [17]. In 1996, Satarug et al. done an interesting study to examine in vivo the activity of cytochrome P450 (CYP) 2A6, an enzyme capable of activating carcinogens, including N-nitrosodimethylamine, in human beings with the carcinogenic liver fluke infection, opisthorchiasis viverrini, before and after therapy with the antiparasitic agent, praziquantel [18]. According to this study, Satarug et al. noted that the expand in CYP 2A6-related enzyme activity might represent an important mechanistic connect between inflammatory products of chronic liver fluke infection, including DNA alkylation damage from endogenously formed N-nitrosamines, and the high risk of cholangiocarcinoma faced by infected individuals [18]. Concerning the molecular biology of opisthorchiasis, Wongratanacheewin et al. saoi that the genome of *O. viverrini* poses neither CpG nor A methylated as found in other parasitic organisms and the total length *O. viverrini* ribosomal DNA is approximately 13 kb. and the existence of a highly repeated DNA specific for the parasitic organism was demonstrated [19]. Recently, Wongratanachewin et al. developed a PCR mean using a pair of primers named OV-6F/OV-6R for detecting *O. viverrini* eggs in stool samples and compared it with Stoll's egg-count mean. In this work, the primers were designed based on the pOV-A6 specific DNA probe sequence which gave a 330 base pair product [20]. They reported that this PCR mean could detect a sole egg in artificially inoculated faeces or as little as 2 x 10(-17) ng of *O. viverrini* genomic DNA [20]. In 2001, Ando et al. compared the mitochondrial cytochrome c oxidase subunit I (CO I) gene and the second internal transcribed spacer region (ITS II) gene of *O. viverrini* among *O. viverrini* from various settings in northeast Thailand [21]. They found that nucleotide sequences of partial CO I gene (417 bp) of O. viverrini differed among O. viverrini originated from Ubon Ratana, Leongpleuy, Ban Phai, Maha Sarakham, and Chatturat and these intraspecific variations were classified into 5 patterns but no setting-specific pattem was observed [21]. However, they noted that amino acid sequence deduced from the nucleotide sequences of these genes was identical [21]. They concluded that nucleotide sequences of a region of the O. viverrini ITS II gene (296 bp) from different settings were identic [21].

Pathophysiology and Clinical Presentation

1 Basic Knowledge on the Pathogenic organism

As previously mentioned, *O. viverrini* is the causative agent for opisthorchiasis. Three subspecies of *Bithynia siamensis* and 18 species of cyprinoid fish are susceptible first and second intermediate hosts, respectively [22]. The differentiation between the adult worm of *O. viverrini* and that of the closely related species, *O. felineus* and *Clonorchis sinensis*, is mainly based on the shape and position of the testes and the arrangement of the vitellaria [22]. The morphology of this parasitic organism is similar to that of *O. felineus*, but it poses more deeply lobated testes, situated near the ovary [10]. The appearance and distributed apperance of the vitellaria with few granular clumps and the shorter and wider egg closely resemble that of *C. sinensis* [10]. However, eggs of these flukes are morphologically similar and problematic in detection but the differentiation between opisthorchid and lecithodendrid eggs is possible [22].

Concerning the life cycle of *O. viverrini*, the adult worms live in the biliary system and eggs pass out in feces [10]. On reaching water the eggs are eaten by snails, the first intermediate host [10]. In the snail the miracidia hatch and develop further through the periods of sporocysts, rediae and cercariae in six to eight weeks [10]. The cercariae then leave the snail, penetrate into susceptible fresh water fish, encyst in the muscle and develop into metacercariae, and infective period, in six weeks. When ingested by man or animal the metacercariae excyst in the duodenum or jejunum and then migrate to the bile duct [10]. These become mature within four weeks and begin to create eggs [10]. The life span of the fluke is over 10 years [10]. The snail intermediate hosts are *Bithynia goniomphalus, B. funiculata* and *B. siamensis*. Many species of cyprinoid fish serve as second intermediate host; *Cyclocheilichthys siaja* is the most important [10]. Cats, dogs and many fish ingesting mammals are definitive hosts whereas man and animals acquire infection by ingesting raw fish containing metacercariae cysts. [10]. In Northeast Thailand, "Koi-Pla" is the most popular raw fish dish, leading to liver fluke infestation.

2. Pathophysiology of Liver Fluke Infestation

Liver fluke infestation is a parasitic disease that is caused by the ingestion of contaminated raw fish, the intermediate host. The acute infestation brings no marked clinical symptoms. The fecal egg excretion is consistent and correlate with the worm burden [23]. Although there is no definite association between clinical signs and intensity of infection, not severe hepatomegaly and thickened wall or dilatation of the gallbladder were found more commonly in heavily infected affected cases [23]. Similar to other parasitic infestation, eosinophilia can be observed. Usually, the disease becomes chronic and persists for many years, leading to hepatobiliary disease and cholangiocarcinoma [19]. Less severe presentations include cholangitis, chronic cholecystitis and cholelithiasis [19]. In chronic opisthorchiasis, Beloborodova et al. noted that dysbacteriosis, hypokinesia of the small

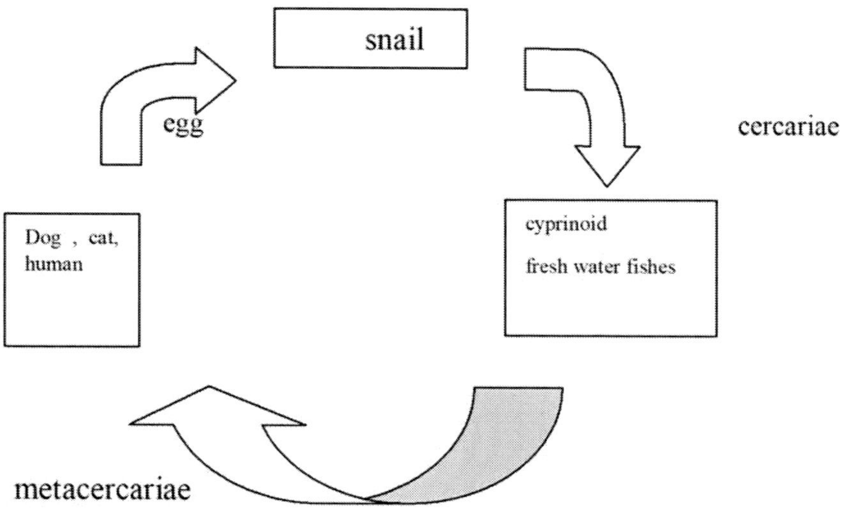

Wiwanitkit V, 2005.

Figure 1. Diagram for life cycle of *O. viverrini.*

intestine, reduction of the cholate-cholesterol ratio of the bile, structural alterations in the small intestine mucosa were found to be implicated in the genesis of malabsorption [24]. They noted that the helminthologic recovery of the affected cases with protracted opisthorchiasis did not entail complete normalization of the function of the small intestine and thus required therapeutic correction [24]. Zvereva et al.said that expanded IgE content was observed mostly in young people in the hypoendemic focus, and in the hyperendemic focus it was in middle-aged and old people, this parameter correlating with decreased levels of gastrin and insulin in the serum [25]. They also noted that gastric basal acid secretion was decreased in more than 70% affected cases from the both groups, however, hyperimmunoglobulinemia tended to show elevated hydrochloric acid debit [25].

Concerning the immune response, a significant degree of humoral and cell mediated immune responses to the parasitic organism can be detected both in affected cases and animal models [19]. The affected cases IgG levels appear to correlate with gall bladder size and dysfunction and correlated significantly with opisthorchis egg count and decrease after therapy [19]. However, the possible importance of these immune responses to protective immunity is presently unknown [19].

3. Clinical Presentation

O. viverrini infection is related with several hepatobiliary diseases including cholangitis, obstructive jaundice, hepatomegaly, cholecystitis and cholelithiasis [2, 26]. Pathological consequences of *O. viverrini* infection occur mainly in the liver, extrahepatic bile ducts, gall bladder and kidney [26]. Moreover, both researchal and epidemiological evidence strongly implicate the liver fluke infection in the etiology of cholangiocarcinoma--the bile duct cancer [2].

Concerning acute opisthorchiasis, cytochemistry was used to study the level of lysosomal cationic proteins of polymorphonuclear peripheral white cells in affected cases with acute and chronic opisthorchiasis, respectively, before therapy [27], suggesting that it was expedient to use lysosomal cationic proteins in combination with other indices for making a diagnosis and determining the period of the disease in Opisthorchis invasion [27]. Similar to other parasitic infestation, eosinophilia in the infected case can be induced by the acute pposese of severe ophisthorchiasis [28]. Concerning the lymphocyte, the acute pposese of opisthorchiasis is characterized by the activation of B lymphocytes and immunological cellular reserve, by depressed T-lymphocytic population with a decreased helper inductor and suppressive killer potential [29]. Kal'gina et al noted that 3 days after dehelminthization, there was a trend for immunoregulatory T cells to become normal and the high levels of B lymphocytes and zero cells were preserved [29]. In 2003, Podkletnova and Stepanova studied the effect of infection rate on parasitic organism-host relations in opisthorchiasis [30].

They noted that the adaptation of the immunity system to recurrent helminth contamination in the natural development of opisthorchiasis accorded with that of the underlying adaptation syndrome in chronic stress [30]. They said that the set correlation makes itself evident in the fact that in recurrent infections with Opisthorchis, the acute (a mobilization pposese) and specifically chronic (a depletion pposese) periods of infestation were characterized by a significant reduction in the overall and specific immunological responsiveness of the host, which was followed by the enhanced biological activity of the parasitic organism [30].

Considering chronic opisthorchiasis, Pungpak et al. studied clinical features of severe opisthorchiasis in 88 affected cases. In this case series, the presenting symptoms were obstructive jaundice, 25% related with secondary infection of biliary system; cholangitis and cholecystitis; intraabdominal mass, which was enlarged liver; 18% had palpable gallbladder; 18% had adenocarcinoma of the bile duct [31]. High bilirubin was found in 46% of scenarioes, high alkaline phosphatase in 80%; elevation of serum transaminase in 78% and low serum albumin in 62% of affected cases [31]. Pungpak et al. noted that there was no correlation between severity of the disease and the fecal egg output [31]. Pungpak et al. said that the obstructive jaundice affected cases had low or no egg output. They also noted that 2 affected cases had no eggs in stool, but numerous *O. viverrini* eggs and flukes were found in the gallbladder and bile ducts at operation [31]. However, Harinasuta et al. reported that the mainity of scenarioes with chronic opisthorchiasis were symptomless [32]. They noted that clinical features varied from not severe to severe and the symptoms and signs included vague gastro-intestinal symptoms, flatulence, anorexia, lassitude, weight loss, dull pain at the right hypochondrium, hot cutaneous sensation of the abdomen, and enlargement of the liver with some tenderness [32]. Harinasuta et al. said that the severe presentations appeared in few scenarioes [32].

Diagnosis of Liver Fluke Infestation

Diagnosis of liver fluke infestation can be done by clinical microscopic technique [1 – 2]. According to the life cycle of the opisthorchiasis, the eggs of parasitic organisms pass into the feces. The characteristics of the *O. viverrini* egg are 22-32 x 11-12 microns in size, light yellowish brown, ovoid body, "electric light bulb" appearance with operculum at the small end and can contain a full developed miracidium [1 – 2] (Figure 2).

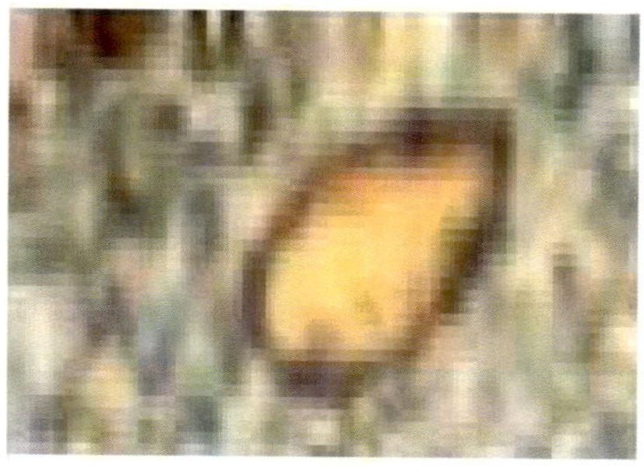

Wiwanitkit V, 2005

Figure 2. Picture of *O. viverrini* egg (X 400, without staining).

Recently, Wiwanitkit and Nithiuthai done an interesting study on the staining mean to help identify of the *O. viverri* eggs [33]. They found that formalin-ether technique help better detect *O. veverrini* eggs [33]. A difficulty in microscopic of *O. viverrni* is the similarity of the *O. viverrini*'s eggs to other minute intestinal fluke egg. In 1999, Sukontason et al. developed a new staining mean for the discrimination between O. viverrini eggs and other similar minute intestinal fluke eggs [34]. In this work, potassium permanganate staining mean was developed for differentiation *O. viverrini*, *Haplorchis taichui* and *Phaneropsolus bonnei* eggs [34]. According to this study, the surfaces of *O. viverrini*, *H. taichui* and *P. bonnei* eggs stained permanently and temporarily were similar in appearance even the staining procedures were varied both in concentration and time [34]. Determined under light microscope set at 400x, all of these eggs were oval-shaped, operculated at one pole and indistinct small knob at posterior end, however, *O. viverrini* eggs showed the distinct musk-melon-like prominent ridges on the surface, *H. taichui* eggs had a light striae pattern whereas *P. bonnei* eggs had a smooth egg shell [34]. In addition, length of these trematode eggs were significant different [34]. Sukontason et al. proposed that temporary staining using 1% w/v concentration and only 1 minute of time was useful in the mass fecal examination survey for the prevalence and intensity of truly Opisthorchis infection [34]. Although difficulty in microscopic diagnosis is the similarity between liver fluke eggs and intestinal fluke eggs the drug of choice is similar.

The immunological diagnosis is not a useful alternative diagnostic technique. The roles of immunological investigation for opisthorchiasis is limited. The development of immunodiagnostic mean for *O. viverrini* detection poses been attempted [19]. The components with molecular weight >116, 89, 78 and 20 kDa appear to be specifically related with the somatic extract of adult fluke [19]. The 89 kDa protein is the most prominent component found in the in vitro culture fluid of adult worms and the metacercarial extract that can be a candidate with significant immunodiagnostic potential [19]. To differentiate between liver fluke and intestinal fluke, the ELISA might be useful in this category. ELISA is often used for the detection of *O.viverrini*-specific antigens (coproantigens) and antibodies (IgM, IgG, IgA, or IgE) [35]. Highly specific and sensitive monoclonal antibodies for O. viverrini antigens were prepared to detect parasitic organism antigens in stool and antibody in serum [19]. Monoclonal antibodies are prepared to detect coproantigens, whereas the crude somatic and excretory-secretory antigens from the adult worms, metacercariae, eggs, and snail intermediate hosts are prepared in order to detect antibodies in sera [35].

In 1987, a study was conducted to determine the value of peritoneoscopy in the diagnosis of opisthorchiasis [36]. In this work peritoneoscopic findings in 203 proven scenarioes of *O. viverrini* infection were studied [36]. Hitanant et al. found that cholangiocarcinoma is commonly encountered in affected cases presenting with prolonged jaundice and hepatomegaly as well as with the peritoneoscopic findings of dilated superficial intrahepatic bile ducts, a bile-stained liver surface and a markedly enlarged gallbladder [36].

Pathology and Complication

For liver fluke infestation, the pathological changes are more or less related to the intensity and the duration of the infection, and are commonly seen in older affected cases with a large number of flukes [32]. Harinasuta et al. said that the pathogenic organismesis was owing to the mechanical irritation by the flukes and some toxic substances created by them and problematic lesions were mainly confined to the biliary system [32]. Harinasuta et al. noted that there was hyperplasia of the epithelial cells lining the bile ducts [32].

Thuwajit et al. recently proposed that, in addition to the direct damage of the bile duct epithelium via direct contact with *O. viverrini*, the excretory/secretory (ES) product(s) released from the parasitic organisms might play important roles in this process [37]. Thuwajit et al investigated the responses of a fibroblast cell line, NIH-3T3, to ES product(s) released from *O. viverrini* by using a non-contact co-culture technique [37]. According to this work, the results indicated a marked expand in NIH-3T3 cell proliferation in the non-contact co-culture condition with either 0% or 10% calf serum in the medium compared with one without parasitic organisms and ES product(s) expanded cell proliferation by stimulating the expression of phosphorylated retinoblastoma (pRB) and cyclin D1, the key proteins in driving cells through the G1/S transition point of the cell cycle [37]. Thuwajit et al. mentioned that this led to the induction of cells going into the S-pposese of the cell cycle. ES product(s) also changed the morphology of NIH-3T3 cells to a refractive and narrow shape, which permited the cells to proliferate in the limited culture setting [37]. In this work, Thuwajit et al. had been able to demonstrate expanded cell proliferation induced by the ES product(s) from O. viverrini and this finding might clarify how *O. viverrini* ES product(s) affect human bile duct epithelium during cholangiocarcinogenesis [37].

In heavy and severe infections there are obstruction of the biliary tract, bile retention, extensive hyperplasia of the biliary system, with glandular proliferation of papillomatous and adenomatous type, cholangitis, periductal infiltration with eosinophils, round cells and fibrosis in the portal settings, necrosis and atrophy of hepatic cells [32]. The bile ducts are dilated and in late scenarioes saccular or cystic formations might develop into large cysts [32]. The gallbladder might enlarge and contain white bile [32]. Considering the biochemical change, the liver profile is generally normal [32]. Concerning the complication of opisthorchiais, there is relapsing cholangitis, the affected case is seriously ill and might succumb to septic shock [32]. Brazhnikova et al. noted that purulent cholangitis was found in about 45 % of the affected cases operated on for complicated forms of opisthorchiasis [38]. They noted that mechanical cholestasis owing to sclerotic changes in the bile ducts, main duodenal papilla and pancreas is the most responsible factor in disease prognosis [38].

Brazhnikova et al .noted that the acute form of purulent cholangitis was attended by acute liver insufficiency in 42.4 per cent of the scenarioes and fatal outcomes took place in 8.2 per cent [38]. They proposed that cholecystectomy had to be supplemented by the restoration of passage of bile in the duodenum with external drainage of the bile ducts to eliminate bacterial flora and helminths [38].

Cholangiocarcinoma, gallstones and obstructive jaundice are not unusual associations [32]. Sripa et al. said that biliary stones were commonly encountered in settings endemic for opisthorchiasis in Thailand [39]. Recently, Sripa et al. done an interesting study on the opisthochiasis-related gall stone diseases [39]. In this work, gallstones and/or common bile duct stones and bile specimens from 113 consecutive cholecystectomies were included and bile samples, including sludge and/or microcalculi, were examined for Opisthorchis viverrini eggs, calcium and bilirubin [39]. In addition, the stones were also processed for scanning electron microscopic (SEM) study [39]. According to this study, bile examination was positive for *O. viverrini* eggs in 50% of the scenarioes studied and aggregates of calcium bilirubinate precipitates were observed in all scenarioes with sludge [39]. In addition, deposition of calcium bilirubinate on the eggshell was visualized by special staining and A SEM study demonstrated the existence of the parasitic organism eggs in the stones [39]. Sripa et al concluded that liver fluke infestation seemed involved in the pathogenic organismesis of stone formation [39].

Severe complications of human liver fluke infestation can be seen in the scenarioes with development of cancer of biliary duct. Mortality is the most serious outcome and usually relate with the cholangiocarcinoma. To clarify the mechanism of carcinogenesis induced by repeated *O.viverrini* infection, Pinlaor et al. investigated the timehistory of 8-nitroguanine and 8-oxo-7,8-dihydro-2'-deoxyguanosine (8-oxodG) formation, inducible nitric oxide syntposese (iNOS) expression, nitric oxide generation and pathological features in hamsters with two (2-IF) or three (3-IF) *O.viverrini* infections [40]. In this study, proliferating cell nuclear antigen accumulated in the epithelium of bile ducts on day 90 after repeated *O.viverrini* infection, supporting the hypothesis that cell proliferation was promoted by inflammation-mediated DNA damage [40]. Conclusively, more common *O. viverrini* infection can induce the expression of iNOS not only in inflammatory cells but also in the epithelium of bile ducts and subsequently cause nitrosative and oxidative damage to nucleic acids, which might participate in the initiation and/or promotion steps of cholangiocarcinoma development [40].

Therapy

For liver fluke infestation, praziquantel is the classical drug. The recommended dose of praziquantel for the therapy and control of opisthorchiasis in the endemic setting is a sole dose of 40 mg per kg body weight after meals [41].

According to the clinical trial of praziquantel, side reactions included headache, dizziness, myalgia and lassitude: however, no laboratory evidence of toxicity was detected [42]. Considering the effect of praziquantel on the fluke, analyses of the surface teguments of flukes exposed to praziquantel either in vitro or in vivo showed similar changes [43]. Sirisinha et al. noted that tegumental bubbles of different sizes appeared on the surface; they later ruptured and resulted in the formation of crater-like problematic lesions and these problematic lesions might be so extensive as to result in the peeling of the entire settings [43]. On occasions, "micronodules" appeared later in these settings and those at the periphery of the problematic lesions; these micronodules might represent an attempt by the worm to regenerate new tegument [43]. Sirisinha et al. said that the possibility that these ultrastructural changes might represent generalized response of the tegumental surface to an obnoxious agent [43]. Recently, the effects of praziquantel coupled with dehydroepiandrosterone (DHEA) or butylated hydroxyanisole (BHA) administration 16 weeks subsequent to dihydroxy-di-n-propylnitrosamine (DHPN) therapy and infection with *O. viverrini* on problematic lesion development in the liver of Syrian hamsters were investigated [44]. According to this study, histopathological assessment revealed that, whereas antihelminthic therapy alone resulted in a clear reduction in hepatocellular problematic lesion development, effects on cholangiocellular problematic lesions were equivocal and BHA and DHEA, in contrast, were both related with a significant reduction in frequency of cholangiofibrosis and cholangiocellular carcinoma [44]. The results thus indicate that although cholangiocellular problematic lesion development might, unlike generation of hepatocellular nodules, be, to a certain extent, independent of the continued existence of parasitic organism, it can be influenced by exogenous therapys [44]. Bakshtanovskaia et al said that pathogenic organismetic therapy was found to alleviate an acute inflammatory process in the liver, but without eliminating cholestasis completely [45]. They noted that antihelminthic therapy improved the results of hepatic tests in different periods after therapy for acute or chronic opisthorchiasis in relation to the rate of compensation of structural problematic lesions [45].

Prevention

Prevention of the liver fluke infestation can be easily done based on the principle of basic food sanitation. The deep-rooted habit of ingestion of raw and poorly uncooked fresh water fishes should be corrected. Similar to gnathostomiasis, health education is needed. Jongsuksuntigul and Imsomboon noted that the main strategies for liver fluke control comprised of three interrelated approaches, namely stool examinations and therapy of positive scenarioes with praziquantel for eliminating human host reservoir; health education for a promotion of cooked fish consumption to prevent infection, and the improvement of hygienic defecation for the interruption of disease transmission [46]. It is accepted that most sucessful is a plan that integrates parasitic organism control, environmental management, health education, and food no danger [16]. Sithithaworn et al. noted that the optimal time for large-scale community-based parasitic organism control plans was when the probability of rapid reinfection was lowest and the prevalence and intensity of infection in people were highest, the summer months [16].

Surveillance of the contamination of the metacercariae in the fresh water intermediate hosts is also important preventive mean. There are many epidemiological investigations on the contamination of the metacercariae in the fresh water intermediate hosts in many endemic countries. The results can be the indicator for the successful of the control plan. Owing to the recent study of Nithiuthai et al. the prevelence of metacercariae in the fresh water fishes in the endemic setting of opisthorchiasis with mass distributed apperance of praziquantel and opisthorchiasis control plan in Thailand revealed null prevalence of *O. viverrrini* metacercariae [47].

Non *Opisthorchis Viverrini* Liver Fluke Infestations

In additional to *O. viverrini* infestation, there are also other liver fluke infestations. Clonochiasis, another infestation caused by *Clonorchis sinensis*, is another widely mentioned liver fluke infestation. The endemic setting of this disease, however, is not actual tropical setting but temperate setting in Eastern Asia [48]. The oriental liverfluke, *C. sinensis*, is of main socioeconomic importance in parts of Asia, including China, Japan, Korea and Taiwan [48]. Similar to *O. viverrini*, the parasitic organism is transmitted via snails to freshwater fish, and then to human beings and other piscivorous mammals, and causes substantial clinical or subclinical disease, known as clonorchiasis [48]. There is also considerable evidence for an etiological relation between clonorchiasis and cholangiocarcinoma in human beings [48]. Clonorchiasis induces biliary epithelial hyperplasia and metaplasia, and this could facilitate at least one period of the carcinogenesis, which is promoting effect [49]. It is estimated that about 35 million people are infected globally, of whom approximately 15 million are in China [48]. It is suggested that clonorchiasis is having an expanded human-health impact owing to the greater consumption of raw freshwater fish [48].

O. felinius infestation is another important liver fluke infestation. Indeed, this parasitic organism is not the specific species for human but cat. Human infestation is sporadic [50 – 51]. The endemic settings include not only tropical but also other settings including Siberia and the Ukraine. Cherdron and Fiegel P said that this cat liver fluke should be added into the differential diagnosis of right-side upper abdominal pain [50].

References

[1] Mairiang E, Mairiang P. Clinical presentation of opisthorchiasis and therapy. *Acta Trop.* 2003;88:221-7.

[2] Sripa B. Pathobiology of opisthorchiasis: an update. *Acta Trop.* 2003;88:209-20.

[3] Wongratanacheewin S, Sermswan RW, Sirisinha S. Immunology and molecular biology of Opisthorchis viverrini infection. *Acta Trop.* 2003;88:195-207.

[4] Upatham ES, Viyanant V. Opisthorchis viverrini and opisthorchiasis: a historical review and future perspective. *Acta Trop.* 2003;88:171-6.

[5] Stauffer WM, Sellman JS, Walker PF. Biliary liver flukes (Opisthorchiasis and Clonorchiasis) in immigrants in the United States: often subtle and diagnosed years after arrival. *J. Travel Med.* 2004 ;11:157-9.

[6] Wiwanitkit V, Suwansaksri J, Chaiyakhun Y. High prevalence of Fasciolopsis buski in an endemic setting of liver fluke infection in Thailand. MedGenMed. 2002;4:6.

[7] Wiwanitkit V. Clinical findings among 62 Thais with cholangiocarcinoma.Trop. Med. Int. Health 2003;8:228-30.

[8] Wiwanitkit V. High serum alkaline phosphatase levels, a study in 181 Thai adult hospitalized affected cases. BMC Fam Pract 2001;2:2.

[9] Sithithaworn P, poseswell-Elkins M. Epidemiology of Opisthorchis viverrini. Acta Trop. 2003;88:187-94.

[10] Harinasuta C, Harinasuta T. Opisthorchis viverrini: life cycle, intermediate hosts, transmission to man and geographical distributed apperance in Thailand. Arzneimittelforschung. 1984;34:1164-7.

[11] Sriamporn S, Pisani P, Pipitgool V, Suwanrungruang K, Kamsa-ard S, Parkin DM. Prevalence of Opisthorchis viverrini infection and incident rate of cholangiocarcinoma in Khon Kaen, Northeast Thailand. *Trop Med Int Health.* 2004;9:588-94.

[12] Yossepowitch O, Gotesman T, Assous M, Marva E, Zimlichman R, Dan M. Opisthorchiasis from imported raw fish. Emerg Infect Dis. 2004;10:2122-6.

[13] Cheng HS, Shieh YH. Investigation on subclinical aspects related to intestinal parasitic infections among Thai laborers in Taipei. *J Travel Med.* 2000;7:319-24.

[14] Saksirisampant W, Wiwanitkit V, Akrabovorn P, Nuchprayoon S. Parasitic infections in Thai workers that pursue overseas employment: the requirement for a screening plan. *Southeast Asian J. Trop. Med. Public Health.* 2002;33 Suppl 3:110-2.

[15] Waikagul J. Opisthorchis viverrini metacercaria in Thai freshwater fish. *Southeast Asian J. Trop. Med. Public Health.* 1998;29:324-6.

[16] Sithithaworn P, Pipitgool V, Srisawangwong T, Elkins DB, Poseswell-Elkins MR. Seasonal variation of Opisthorchis viverrini infection in cyprinoid fish in north-east Thailand: implications for parasitic organism control and food no danger. *Bull. World Health Organ.* 1997;75:125-31.

[17] Honjo S, Srivatanakul P, Sriplung H, Kikukawa H, Hanai S, Uchida K, Todoroki T, Jedpiyawongse A, Kittiwatanachot P, Sripa B, Deerasamee S, Miwa M. Genetic and environmental determinants of risk for cholangiocarcinoma via Opisthorchis viverrini in a densely infested setting in Nakhon Phanom, northeast *Thailand. Int J. Cancer.* 2005

[18] Satarug S, Lang MA, Yongvanit P, Sithithaworn P, Mairiang E, Mairiang P, Pelkonen P, Bartsch H, Poseswell-Elkins MR. Induction of cytochrome P450 2A6 expression in human beings by the carcinogenic parasitic organism infection, opisthorchiasis viverrini. *Cancer Epidemiol. Biomarkers Prev.* 1996;5:795-800.

[19] Wongratanacheewin S, Sermswan RW, Sirisinha S. Immunology and molecular biology of Opisthorchis viverrini infection. *Acta Trop.* 2003;88:195-207.

[20] Wongratanacheewin S, Pumidonming W, Sermswan RW, Maleewong W. Development of a PCR-based mean for the detection of Opisthorchis viverrini in researchally infected hamsters. *Parasitology.* 2001;122:175-80.

[21] Ando K, Sithithaworn P, Nuchjungreed C, Tesana S, Srisawangwong T, Limviroj W, Chinzei Y. Nucleotide sequence of mitochondrial CO I and ribosomal ITS II genes of Opisthorchis viverrini in northeast Thailand. *Southeast Asian J. Trop. Med. Public Health.* 2001;32 Suppl 2:17-22.

[22] Kaewkes S. Taxonomy and biology of liver flukes. *Acta Trop.* 2003;88:177-86.

[23] Pungpak S, Harinasuta T, Bunnag D, Chindanond D, Radomyos P. Fecal egg output in relation to worm burden and clinical features in human opisthorchiasis. *Southeast Asian J. Trop .Med. Public Health.* 1990;21:275-80.

[24] Beloborodova EI, Kaliuzhina MI, Soldatova LP. Clinico-functional status of the small intestine in affected cases with chronic opisthorchiasis. *Ter Arkh.* 1989;61:64-7.

[25] Zvereva LI, Mamin VV, Kopytov II, Kortev AI, Ozeretskovskaia NN. The secretory activity of the stomach, duodenum and pancreas in affected cases with chronic opisthorchiasis. *Med. Parazitol* (Mosk). 1989;(5):17-21.

[26] Mairiang E, Mairiang P. Clinical presentation of opisthorchiasis and therapy. *Acta Trop.* 2003;88:221-7.

[27] Iakovleva VV, Stepanova TF, Androsova EV, Postnikova TF, Shonin AL. Expand of lysosomal cationic proteins of polymorphonuclear white cells as a response to opisthorchis invasion. *Med. Parazitol* (Mosk). 2003;(2):7-10.

[28] Nishiura H, Tsunoda T, Akao N. A case of severe eosinophilia in the acute pposese of Opisthorchis viverrini infection. Kansenshogaku Zasshi. 2003;77:677-81.

[29] Kal'gina GA, Stepanova TF, Shonin AL. The populational structure of peripheral lymphocytes in affected cases in the acute pposese of opisthorchiasis. *Med. Parazitol* (Mosk). 2002;(1):16-8.

[30] Podkletnova LF, Stepanova TF. Effect of infection rate on parasitic organism-host relations in opisthorchiasis. *Med. Parazitol* (Mosk). 2003;(1):16-21.

[31] Pungpak S, Riganti M, Bunnag D, Harinasuta T. Clinical features in severe opisthorchiasis viverrini. *Southeast Asian J Trop Med Public Health.* 1985 ;16:405-9.

[32] Harinasuta T, Riganti M, Bunnag D. Opisthorchis viverrini infection: pathogenic organismesis and clinical features. Arzneimittelforschung. 1984;34:1167-9.

[33] Wiwanitkit V, Nithiuthai S. Which is better for detection of Opisthorchis viverrini eggs: simple smear and formalin-ether technique. Infect Dis Antimicrob Agent 2002; 19: 6 – 8.

[34] Sukontason K, Piangjai S, Sukontason K, Chaithong U. Potassium permanganate staining for differentiation the surface morphology of Opisthorchis viverrini, Haplorchis taichui and Phaneropsolus bonnei eggs. *Southeast Asian J. Trop. Med. Public Health.* 1999;30:371-4.

[35] Jamornthanyawat N. The diagnosis of human opisthorchiasis. Southeast Asian J. Trop Med. Public Health. 2002;33 Suppl 3:86-91.

[36] Hitanant S, Trong DT, Damrongsak C, Chinapak O, Boonyapisit S, Plengvanit U, Viranuvatti V. Peritoneoscopic findings in 203 affected cases with Opisthorchis viverrini infection. *Gastrointest Endosc.* 1987;33:18-20.

[37] Thuwajit C, Thuwajit P, Kaewkes S, Sripa B, Uchida K, Miwa M, Wongkham S. Expanded cell proliferation of mouse fibroblast NIH-3T3 in vitro induced by excretory/secretory product(s) from Opisthorchis viverrini. *Parasitology.* 2004 ;129:455-64.

[38] Brazhnikova NA. Opisthorchiasis-induced suppurative cholangitis (clinical history and diagnosis). *Klin. Med* (Mosk). 1989;67:89-94.

[39] Sripa B, Kanla P, Sinawat P, Poseswell-Elkins MR. Opisthorchiasis-related biliary stones: light and scanning electron microscopic study. *World J. Gastroenterol.* 2004;10:3318-21.

[40] Pinlaor S, Ma N, Hiraku Y, Yongvanit P, Semba R, Oikawa S, Murata M, Sripa B, Sithithaworn P, Kawanishi S. Repeated infection with Opisthorchis viverrini induces accumulation of 8-nitroguanine and 8-oxo-7,8-dihydro-2'-deoxyguanine in the bile duct of hamsters via inducible nitric oxide syntposese. Carcinogenesis. 2004;25:1535-42.

[41] Bunnag D, Harinasuta T. Studies on the chemotherapy of human opisthorchiasis: III. Minimum sucessful dose of praziquantel. *Southeast Asian J. Trop. Med. Public Health.* 1981;12:413-7.

[42] Bunnag D, Harinasuta T. Studies on the chemotherapy of human opisthorchiasis in Thailand: I. Clinical trial of praziquantel. *Southeast Asian J. Trop. Med. Public Health.* 1980;11:528-31.

[43] Sirisinha S, Puengtomwatanakul S, Sobhon P, Saitongdee P, Wongpayabal P, Mitranonde V, Radomyos P, Bunnag D, Harinasuta T. Alterations of the surface tegument of Opisthorchis viverrini exposed to praziquantel in vitro and in vivo. *Southeast Asian J. Trop. Med. Public Health.* 1984;15:95-103.

[44] Moore MA, Thamavit W, Tiwawech D, Ito N, Tsuda H.Modulation of dihydroxy-di-n-propylnitrosamine-induced liver problematic lesion development in Opisthorchis-infected Syrian hamsters by praziquantel therapy in ssociation with butylated hydroxyanisole or dehydroepiandrosterone administration. *Jpn. J. Cancer Res.* 1998;89:1113-7.

[45] Bakshtanovskaia IV, Stepanova TF, Shonin AL, Ponomareva OV, Terekhina VK, Kholodkovskaia NV. Impact of anthelminthic therapy for opisthorchiasis on the biochemical parameters of hepatic function. Med Parazitol (Mosk). 2003;(2):10-5.

[46] Jongsuksuntigul P, Imsomboon T. Opisthorchiasis control in Thailand. *Acta Trop.* 2003;88:229-32.

[47] Nithiuthai S, Suwansaksri J, Wiwanitkit V, Chaengphukeaw P. A survey of metacercariae in cyprinoid fish in Nakhon Ratcposesima, northeast Thailand. *Southeast Asian J. Trop. Med. Public Health.* 2002;33 Suppl 3:103-5.

[48] Lun ZR, Gasser RB, Lai DH, Li AX, Zhu XQ, Yu XB, Fang YY. Clonorchiasis: a key foodborne zoonosis in China. *Lancet Infect Dis.* 2005;5:31-41.

[49] Choi BI, Han JK, Hong ST, Lee KH. Clonorchiasis and cholangiocarcinoma: etiologic relationship and imaging diagnosis. *Clin. Microbiol. Rev.* 2004;17:540-52.

[50] Cherdron A, Fiegel P. Opisthorchis felineus--the cat liver fluke. Differential diagnosis of right-side upper abdominal pain. Dtsch Med Wochenschr. 1992;117:328-31.

[51] Tselepatiotis E, Mantadakis E, Papoulis S, Vassalou E, Kotsakis P, Samonis G.A case of Opisthorchis felineus infestation in a pilot from Greece.*Infection.* 2003;31:430-2.

Chapter 4

Fluke Infestation 2: Echinostomiasis And Other Minute Intestinal Fluke Infestation

Echinostomiasis

A. Introduction to Echinostomiasis

Echinostomiasis is an helminthic zoonotic disease. Human echinostomiasis, endemic to southeast Asia and the Far East, is a food-borne, intestinal, zoonotic parasitosis attributed to at least 16 species of digenean trematodes transmitted by snails [1]. Numerous echinostome trematodes are found in the intestines of birds and mammals throughout the world [2]. Two separate life cycles of echinostomes, human and sylvatic, efficiently operate in endemic settings [1].

Echinostomiasis is aggravated by socioeconomic factors including poverty, malnutrition, an explosively growing free-food market, a lack of supervised food inspection, poor or insufficient sanitation, other helminthiases, and declining economic conditions [1]. Prevention of human scenarioes is dependent on ingesting habits, since raw or insufficiently cooked molluses, and to a lesser extent fish and amphibians, are sources of infection for human beings [2]. Human scenarioes pose been sucessfully, albeit accidentally, controlled by the introduction of fish which prey on the larval periods of the essential molluscan hosts[2]. Furthermore, World Health Organization control plans implemented for other food-borne helminthiases and sustained in endemic settings are not fully successful for echinostomiasis because these parasitic organisms display extremely broad specificity for the second intermediate host and are capable of completing the life cycle without involvement of the human host [1].

B. Epidemiology of Echinostomiasis

The prevalence of infection ranges from 44% in the Philippines to 5% in mainland China, and from 50% in northern Thailand to 9% in Korea [1]. Although the patterns of other food-borne trematodiases pose changed in Asia following changes in habits, cultural practices, health education, industrialization, and environmental alteration, human echinostomiasis remains a health problem [1]. The disease is most prevalent in remote rural places among low-wage earners and in women of child bearing age [1].

The epidemiological pattern of echinostomiasis caused by different species is believed to relate to the susceptibility of the intermediate host. DeGaffe and Loker said that susceptibility of the snail *Biomphalaria glabrata* to infection with the digenetic trematode *Echinostoma paraensei* was correlated with the ability of secretory-excretory products (SEP) derived from sporocysts of this parasitic organism to interfere with the spreading behavior of host hemocytes in an in vitro tool [3]. They noted that *E. paraensei* sporocyst SEP effects on host hemocyte spreading mirror observed patterns in both age and strain-related susceptibility of *B. glabrata* to this parasitic organism [3]. The results suggest that the number of hemocytes available to a particular snail influences its vulnerability to infection with *E. paraensei* [3].

Echinostomiasis is rarely reported in travelers, although the disease remains a main public health problem in Southeast Asia. In 1985, Poland et al reported an outbreak of parasitic gastroenteritis among travelers returning from Africa [4]. According to this report, eosinophilia and intestinal infections with a trematode parasitic organism developed in 18 of the 20 American tourists who traveled to Kenya and Tanzania [4]. Several tour members had not severe, nonspecific abdominal complaints, but ten had moderately severe abdominal cramps and loose or watery stools [4]. Because no adult flukes were recovered, a specific detection could not be made, but the eggs we observed resembled those of an Echinostoma [4].

Concerning the effect of environment on the Echinostoma infestation, the seasonal variation of the metacercaria, the infective period larva, is mentioned [5].

A survey of 61 residents belonging to 12 pre-selected families (having at least one member positive for *E malayanum*) from Barangay Malibago, Echague, Isabela (northern Luzon) suggested that infections with *E. malayanum* follow a "familial trend" [5]. In this report, the parasitic organism is endemic because the raw ingestion of *Lymnaea* (*Bullastra*) *cumingiana*, the second intermediate host in the Philippines, is a learned habit passed down from one generation to the next [5]. In addition, a questionnaire on ingesting habits revealed that *L. cumingiana* was usually prepared raw or half-cooked after therapy with salt or salted fish paste [5]. It was abundant in rice fields during the wet months of the year, thus implying a seasonal infection pattern since ingesting frequency was affected by availability [5].

C. Genetic and Molecular Biology of Echinostomiasis

There are some interesting studies concerning the echinostomiasis. In 1995, Sloss et al. done a study on the genetic relationships between *E. caproni*, *E. paraensei*, and *E. trivolvis* as determined by electrophoresis [6]. In this work, adults of *E. caproni*, *E.*

paraensei, and *E. trivolvis* were processed for starch gel electrophoresis and 10 enzyme systems representing 12 structural loci were examined using three different buffer systems [6]. Sloss et al. noted that phenic relationships among the three species showed *E. caproni* was genetically more similar to *E. trivolvis* than to *E. paraensei* [6]. Fujino et al done a similar study, a comparison of *E. trivolvis* and *E. caproni* using random amplified polymorphic DNA analysis, in 1995 [7]. According to this study, band patterns generated using five individual primers showed that these two echinostomes were genetically distinct, although they share genomic DNA to some extent [7].

Snail immune responses towards a trematode infection are known to rely on both plasmatic and cellular host factors [8 – 9]. The sporocyst period of trematode development plays the crucial role of establishing a successful infection in the molluscan intermediate host [8]. Owing to the small size and existence of this period within the tissues of the host, much of current knowledge of sporocyst biology relies on cultured specimens [8]. In 2005, Nowak and Loger done an interesting study to gain insight into the transcriptional patterns of early sporocysts, suppression subtractive hybridization was employed to identify 69 unique expressed sequence tags likely to be upregulated in cultured sporocysts of *E. paraensei*, a trematode parasitic organism of the planorbid snail, *B. glabrata* [8]. In this work, upwards of 70% of the unique sequences were not identified by homology to known genes [8]. As an approach to further investigate the suspected involvement of plasmatic factors in *B. glabrata* resistance/susceptibility to *E. caproni*, Vergote et al. compared protein patterns of plasma collected from susceptible and resistant snails [9]. This study showed that: (a) differential representation of plasma proteins between the snail strains was correlated with a differential level of transcripts; (b) expression of these genes after parasitic organism exposure was differentially regulated in the two strains; and (c) these genes were expressed predominantly in the albumen gland [9].

D. Pathophysiology and Clinical Presentation

1 Basic Knowledge on the Pathogenic organism

Human echinostomiasis is caused by digenetic trematodes of the genus Echinostoma. Concerning the life cycle of Ehinostoma, The complex life cycles of echinostomes are all connected to freshwater habitats [2]. A mammalian or avian definitive host, one or two molluscan hosts, and one or two freshwater periods are usually required to complete the life cycle [2]. In addition, amphibians and fish pose been implicated in the transmission of some species [2]. Ataev et al. said that Echinostomatidae is intermediate between two groups of trematodes [10]. They noted that the first group had mother sporocyst (MS) that completely realize reproductive function in the time of miracidial formation; but the second group included higher trematodes characterized by the transfer of reproductive time on a parasitic pposese of MS development [10]. The disease occurs focally and transmission is connected to fresh or brackish water habitats [1]. Infections are related with common sociocultural practices of ingesting raw or insufficiently cooked mollusks, fish, crustaceans, and amphibians, promiscuous defecation, and the use of night soil (human excrement collected from latrines) for fertilization of fish ponds [1].

2. Pathophysiology of Echinostomiasis

There are some interesting studies on the pathophysiology of echinostomiasis.

In 1997, infectivity and growth studies in domestic chicks were carried out on a strain of *E. revolutum* isolated from Lymnaea elodes snails in Indiana, USA by Humphries et al [11]. Humphries et al. said that growth of *E. revolutum* in the chick was delayed compared to previous findings on *E. trivolvis*, a closely related species of 37-collar-spined echinostome in the *E. revolutum* complex [11]. In 1995, Kaufman and Fried et al. showed how that short-duration removal of food had no effect on worm survival, size or distributed apperance of *E. caproni* adults in the small intestine of the ICR mouse [12]. In 1991, Bindseil and Hau et al. proposed that infection in mice with the intestinal trematode Echinostoma caproni had a negative influence on pregnancy [13]. In their study, the effect of the infection set in immediately following implantation (day 5 of pregnancy) resulting in fewer fetuses being present in infected mice on day 9 than in the controls, however, Ovulation, fertilization of eggs, and implantation itself were obviously not impaired [13]. In addition, the infected mice had significantly lower serum progesterone levels on day 5 of pregnancy than the non-infected controls [13]. According to this study, it is speculated that the progesterone levels in the infected female mice were too low to secure early post-implantation gestation [13].

3. Clinical Presentation

Clinical symptoms of echinostomiasis include abdominal pain, violent watery diarrhea, and anorexia [1]. In human beings it is usually regarded as a rare intestinal parasitic organism of little clinical importance except in heavy infections [2]. In the heavy infection scenarioes, the abdominal pain is the common presentation.

E. Diagnosis of Echinostomiasis

Diagnosis of echinostomiasis is made by detection of eggs during fecal examination; however, speciation of echinostomes requires morphological study of adult worms following anthelminthic therapy [2]. Occasionally endoscopy is useful in diagnosis of echinostomiasis [14 – 16]. Chang et al. reported a Korean woman, who had history of ingesting raw frog meat, presented at a local clinic with complaints of abdominal pain and discomfort that had persisted for 2 weeks [14]. Under gastroduodenoscopy, two motile flukes were found attached on the duodenal bulb, and retrieved with endoscopic forceps [14]. Finally, the two flukes were identified as *E. hortense* by egg morphology, 27 collar spines with 4 end-group spines, and surface ultrastructural characters [14]. Another Korean male, in the habit of ingesting fresh water fish, living in Yeongcheon-shi, Gyeongsangbuk-do and with epigastric discomfort of several days duration, was subjected to upper gastrointestinal endoscopy [15]. In this case, 2 live worms were found in the duodenal bulb setting and were removed using an endoscopic forceps and the worms were identified as *E. hortense* based on their morphological characteristics [15].

The roles of immunological investigation for echnostomiasis is limited. In 1994, Graczyk and Fried set an ELISA mean for detecting anti-*E. caproni* immunoglobulins in researchally infected ICR mice [17]. In this work, an utilizing surface glycocalyx membrane crude antigen of adult *E. caproni* was developed for the detection of circulating anti-*E. caproni* immunoglobulins in sera from researchally infected ICR mice [17]. Graczyk and Fried found that whole blood, serum, and dried blood on filter paper gave similar results but the latter was selected for convenience [17].

F.Pathology and Complication

Huffman et al. done an interesting animal research in 1986 [18]. In this work, clinical and pathological effects of *E. revolutum* in the golden hamster, *Mesocricetus auratus* was studied [18]. Clinical signs included progressive unthriftiness, watery diarrhea and weight loss [18]. Packed cell volume, hemoglobin and red blood cell counts expanded in those animals with severe diarrhea [18]. No expand in eosinophils was noted in peripheral blood smears [18]. Examination of tissues of infected animals showed wide individual variations related to the intensity of infection [18]. The histopathological responses of hamsters to the parasitic organism showed erosion of intestinal villi with lymphocytic infiltration being the primary response[18]. Periportal lymphocytic infiltration and focal hepatic necrosis were observed in livers from some infected animals [18].

In 1993, Fujino et al. done a similar animal researchal study on the expulsion of *E. trivolvis* focusing at worm kinetics and intestinal cytopathology in conventional and congenitally athymic BALB/c mice [19]. According to this study, whereas common pathological changes occurred in the intestines of both mice groups infected with echinostomes some ultrastructural differences were observed in the intestine epithelial cells of conventional versus athymic mice [19]. In 1993, Fujino and Fried found that *E. caproni* and *E. trivolvis* could alter the binding of glycoconjugates in the intestinal mucosa of C3H mice as determined by lectin histochemistry [20]. In 1993, Fujino and Fried also studied the expulsion of *E. trivolvis* and retention of *E. caproni*in C3H mice for pathological, ultrastructural, and cytochemical effects on the host intestine [21]. In mice infected with *E. caproni*, the intestine showed villous atrophy with fused or eroded villi [21]. The microvilli of the enterocytes were sparse and distorted and showed minimized alkaline phosphatase activity [21]. The crypts of Lieberkuhn were hyperplastic and showed a marked reduction in goblet and Paneth cells [21]. As compared with uninfected controls, there was a marked reduction in glucose-6-phosphatase activity in the enterocytes of the infected intestine [21]. Collagen fibers and the number of fibroblasts were expanded under the epithelium [21]. In mice infected with *E. trivolvis*, the tips of the intestinal villi were bent and blunted. The microvilli of the enterocytes were less tightly packed than those of uninfected controls [21]. The mitochondria in the enterocytes were irregularly shaped, contained intracristal bodies, and showed expanded cytochrome oxidase activity as compared with those of uninfected controls [21]. The crypts were hyperplastic but showed an expand in the numbers of goblet and Paneth cells [21]. The fibroblasts and collagen fibers showed abnormal development [21].

Lee et al. done an interesting study on chronological observation of intestinal problematic lesions of rats researchally infected with *E. hortense* [22]. In this work, histopathological changes of the intestine were recognizable in as early as 1-3 days after infection, and the changes became severer as the infection progressed [22]. The intestinal mucosa was histopathologically characterized by villous atrophy and crypt hyperplasia throughout the infection period [22]. Main villous changes were blunting, fusion, severe destruction and loss of epithelial layers of villi [22]. In the stroma of villi, inflammatory cell infiltrations, vascular congestion, edema, and/or fibrosis were recognized [22].

Concerning the complication of echinostomiasis, no serious complications in human beings are reported. In 1993, Sanchaisuriya et al. studied nutritional health and parasitic infection of rural Thai women of the child bearing age [23]. They noted that echinostomiasis had no effect on the nutritional status on the infested human [23]. Also, it did not lead to tropical anemia [23].

G. Therapy

For echinostomiasis, praziquantel is the drug of choice [1 – 2]. There are also some reports on the use of other alternative antiparasitic drugs. Maurer et al. recently studied the effects of the anthelmintics clorsulon, rafoxanide, mebendazole and arprinocid on Echinostoma caproni in ICR mice [24]. They found that doses of 100 mg/kg of clorsulon and 50 mg/kg of rafoxanide were 100% sucessful in eliminating the echinostomes on day 1 post-administration of the anthelmintics but mebendazole and arprinocid were insucessful in eliminating worms at 1 or 2 days post drug administration [24].

H. Prevention

Prevention of the echinostomiasis infestation can be easily done based on the principle of basic food sanitation. The deep-rooted habit as ingestion of raw and poorly uncooked foods should be corrected [1 – 2]. Similar to other food-borne zoonoses, health education is needed. Surveillance of the contamination of the metacercariae in the fresh water intermediate hosts is also an important preventive mean. In 1990, Ryang reported the studies on *Echinostoma* spp. in the Chungju Reservoir and upper streams of the Namhan River in Korea [25]. Ryang reported that It poses been proved that the Chungju Reservoir and upper streams of Namhan river are endemic settings of echinostomiasis, especially of *E. hortense*, and snails including *R. auricularia coreana* and fishes including *O. obscura interrupta*, *M. anguillicaudatus*, and others are taking the role of first and second intermediate hosts, respectively [25].

Other Minute Intestinal Fluke Infestations

In additional to Echinostoma, there are also other minute intestinal flukes which can cause the zoonosis infection in human. The details of some important minute intestinal fluke infestations are hereby present:

A. Gymnophalloides Seoi Infection

This minute intestinal fluke, *Gymnophalloides seoi*, was first discovered from a Korean woman suffering from acute pancreatitis and gastrointestinal troubles [26]. Concerning this case, the coastal village where the affected case resided was found to be a highly endemic setting for this fluke, and 24 other endemic settings pose been found [26]. This fluke infection is now recognized as an emerging parasitic disease [26]. Its second intermediate host is the oyster, and migrating birds are a natural definitive host [26]. The parasitic organism is very small, 0.33-0.50 mm long and 0.23-0.33 mm wide, and characterized by the existence of a ventral pit [27]. As previously mentioned, man and the *Palearctic oystercatcher, Haematopus ostralegus* pose been shown to be natural definitive hosts, and wading birds including the *Kentish plover, Charadrius alexandrinus* are highly susceptible to researchal infection [27]. Gerbils, hamsters, cats, and several strains of mice were also susceptible laboratory hosts [27].

Lee and Chai noted that infected people complained of variable degrees of gastrointestinal troubles and indigestion [27]. The infection can be diagnosed by recovery of eggs in the feces; however, an expert is required to identify the eggs [27]. Praziquantel, 10 mg/kg in sole dose, is sucessful for therapy of human infections. Ingesting raw oysters in endemic settings should be avoided [27]. Until present, this species is localized in Korea. Since the endemic setting of this parasitic organism is not an actual tropic setting, the details are hereby given in brief. However, Chai et al said that this new trematode might exist in other countries [26].

B. Haplorchis Taichui Infestation

Haplorchis taichui infestation is another intestinal infection. This species parasitizes the small intestine of human beings and other mammals [28]. In 2005, Sukontason et al presented the pathology in the small intestine of 3 human scenarioes caused by *H. taichui* [28]. Microscopic examination revealed mucosal ulceration, mucosal and submucosal hemorrhages, fusion and shortening villi, chronic inflammation, and fibrosis of the submucosa [28]. Sukontason et al noted that this finding clearly indicated *H. taichui* as pathogenic organismic; thus prevention of infection and therapy should be paramount [28]. The human infection of this parasitic organism is believed to be owing to the ingesting habit of uncooked or poorly cooked fresh water fishes. This infection is endemic in the Southeast Asia. High prevalence of infection (36%) in human beings by *H. taichui* in the Philippines was reported by Belizario et al [29]. Belizario et al said that the likely source of haplorchine infection had been connected to consumption of raw or undercooked freshwater fish containing infective metacercariae [29]. In this series, the most common clinical symptoms appeared as upper abdominal discomfort or pain and borborygmi [29]. In 1991, Giboda et al done a study of the epidemiology of trematode infections was carried out in Vientiane province, Laos, comprising examination of snails, fish, cats, and human stools [30]. According to this study, detection of small flukes excreted by Laotian affected cases after therapy with praziquantel revealed more scenarioes with *H. taichui* than with *Opisthorchis viverrini* [30]. The results confirmed the simultaneous occurrence of *O. viverrini* and intestinal heterophyid flukes in the setting studied [30].

Concerning the therapy, Belizario et al said that praziquantel (75 mg/kg divided in 3 doses in 1 day) was a well-tolerated and sucessful therapy for infection by *H. taichui* [29]. Prevention of the *H. taichui* infestation can be easily done based on the principle of basic food sanitation. The deep-rooted habit as ingestion of raw and poorly uncooked fish dished should be corrected. In 2002, Wiwanitkit et al done a study to examine the motility of Haplorchinae spp metacercariae in matched minnows using a number of preparation means that mimic traditional practices [31]. In this work, 5 different raw fish dishes that mimic traditional meals (2 fishes/dish) were prepared using the following means: 1) left to dry at room temperature; 2) frozen at -20 Celsius; 3) refrigerated at 4 Celsius; 4) marinated in saline (5% sodium chloride solution); and 5) marinated in 5% acetic acid solution to mimic traditional vinegar [31]. According to this study, degeneration of the parasitic organisms was slowed by cooling: degeneration of all metacercariae took approximately 5 hours in the refrigerated or frozen fish, compared with 3 hours in all other dishes left at room temperature [31]. The study substantiates the epidemiologic data demonstrating transmission of these types of pathogenic organisms in spite of freezing, pickling, and salting [31]. Similar to other food-borne zoonoses, health education is needed. Surveillance of the contamination of the metacercariae in the fresh water intermediate hosts is also important preventive mean. Nithiuthai et al recently done a survey of metacercariae in cyprinoid fish in Nakhon Ratcposesima, northeast Thailand [32]. They found that Haplochinae metacercariae were found in all 3 species of fish, giving rates of infection of 95.5%, 20% and 1.9% for *Puntius leiacanthus*, *Cyclocheilichthys armatus* and *Hampla dispar* respectively [32]. This is also the first report of fish infected with Haplorchinae spp in Thailand [32].

C. Heterophyidiasis

Heterophyidiasis is an infection of the small bowel by minute intestinal flukes of the genus Heterophyes or related members of the family Heterophyidae (including *Stellantcposesmus falcatus* infection) [33]. Similar to *H. taichui* infestation, infection had been connected to consumption of raw or undercooked freshwater fish containing infective metacercariae. In 2001, Belizario et al. done a study attempted to determine the infection rate, intensity of infection as well as the clinical spectrum of heterophyid infection [33]. In this study, a stool survey was conducted in barangay San Isidro, Monkayo, Compostela Valley in [33]. Belizario et al. found that 37 % of affected cases with history of bowel disturbance (abdominal discomfort/pain and/or diarrhea) in the past 4 weeks were found to pose heterophyidiasis and prevalence was highest in the 15 to 30 years old group at 55.3% [33]. They noted that the most common clinical presentations of heterophyidiasis were signs and symptoms of acid peptic or peptic ulcer disease [33]. Belizario et al. noted that early diagnosis and therapy were important to ensure prompt resolution of heterophyid infection, hence, decreased morbidity and decreased chances for complications like heart or brain involvement [33]. For therapy, praziquantel is the drug of choice.

Prevention of this infestation is similar to those of *H. taichui*. Uncooked and poorly cooked fish dishes are the important causes of human infection. In 2001, Wiwanitkit et al done a study to examine the motility heterophyid spp metacercariae in matched minnows using a number of preparation means that mimic traditional practices [34]. Similar to the study by Wiwanitkit et al. [31] for the *H. taichui*, this study substantiates the epidemiologic data demonstrating transmission of these types of pathogenic organisms in spite of freezing, pickling, and salting [34].

Surveillance of the contamination of the metacercariae in the fresh water intermediate hosts is also important preventive mean. Nithiuthai et al recently done a survey of metacercariae in cyprinoid fish in Nakhon Ratcposesima, northeast Thailand [32]. They found that Heterophyidae metacercariae were found only in Puntius leiacanthus, whose infection rate was 30.77% [32].

D. Metagonimiasis

Metagonimiasis yokogawai is an intestinal fluke causing metagonimiasis [35].

It is considered as a member of family Heterophyidae. However, since metagonimiasis poses its significant character, it is usually mentioned as a separate disease. The disease cause pathology mainly in the intestine. The small adults trematode of *M. yokogawai* can be found free in jejunal lumen as well as impacted in intervillous spaces [36]. Histologically intestinal problematic lesions include massive lymphoplasmacytic and eosinophilic infiltration in stroma, erosion of neanby enterocytes, goblet cell depletion and occasional villous edema [36]. Scanning electron microscopy can reveal the worm of spatulate appearance with rake-shaped tegumental spines [36]. By transmission electron microscopy, the syncytial integument with dense discoidal bodies, basement membrane muscle cells and subtegumental cells can be observed [36]. Characteristic junctional complex can be demonstrated between subtegumental and parenchymal cells as well as between parenchymal cells [36]. Complications like heart or brain involvement owing to metagonimiasis are mentioned [37]. Since, the endemic setting of this disease is in Japan and Korea, which is not the tropical countries, more details are note hereby presented.

References

[1] Graczyk TK, Fried B. Echinostomiasis: a common but forgotten food-borne disease. Am *J. Trop. Med. Hyg.* 1998;58:501-4.

[2] Carney WP. Echinostomiasis--a snail-borne intestinal trematode zoonosis. *Southeast Asian J. Trop. Med. Public Health.* 1991;22 Suppl:206-11.

[3] DeGaffe G, Loker ES. Susceptibility of Biomphalaria glabrata to infection with Echinostoma paraensei: correlation with the effect of parasitic organism secretory-excretory products on host hemocyte spreading. *J. Invertebr Pathol.* 1998;71:64-72.

[4] Poland GA, Navin TR, Sarosi GA. Outbreak of parasitic gastroenteritis among travelers returning from Africa. *Arch. Intern. Med.* 1985;145:2220-1.

[5] Tangtrongchitr A, Monzon RB. Ingesting habits related with Echinostoma malayanum infections in the Philippines. *Southeast Asian J. Trop. Med. Public Health*. 1991;22 Suppl:212-6.

[6] Sloss B, Meece J, Romano M, Nollen P. The genetic relationships between Echinostoma caproni, E. paraensei, and E. trivolvis as determined by electrophoresis. *J. Helminthol.* 1995;69:243-6.

[7] Fujino T, Takaposeshi Y, Fried B. A comparison of Echinostoma trivolvis and E. caproni using random amplified polymorphic DNA analysis. *J. Helminthol.* 1995 ;69:263-4.

[8] Nowak TS, Loker ES. Echinostoma paraensei: differential gene transcription in the sporocyst period. *Exp. Parasitol.* 2005;109:94-105.

[9] Vergote D, Bouchut A, Sautiere PE, Roger E, Galinier R, Rognon A, Coustau C, Salzet M, Mitta G. Characterisation of proteins differentially present in the plasma of Biomphalaria glabrata susceptible or resistant to Echinostoma caproni. *Int. J. Parasitol.* 2005;35:215-24.

[10] Ataev GL, Avanesian AI, Loker ES, Dobrovol'skii AA. The organization of germinal material and dynamics of mother sporocyst regeneration in the genus Echinostoma (Trematoda: Echinostomatidae). *Parazitologiia*. 2001;35:307-19.

[11] Humphries JE, Reddy A, Fried B. Infectivity and growth of Echinostoma revolutum (Froelich, 1802) in the domestic chick. *Int. J. Parasitol.* 1997;27:129-30.

[12] Kaufman AR, Fried B. The effects of the existence and absence of intestinal contents on survival, size and distributed apperance of Echinostoma caproni in ICR mice. *J. Helminthol.* 1995;69:93-4

[13] Bindseil E, Hau J. Negative effect on early post-implantation pregnancy and progesterone levels in mice infected with the intestinal trematode Echinostoma caproni. *Parasitology*. 1991;102 Pt 3:387-90.

[14] Chang YD, Sohn WM, Ryu JH, Kang SY, Hong SJ. A human infection of Echinostoma hortense in duodenal bulb diagnosed by endoscopy. *Korean J. Parasitol.* 2005;43:57-60.

[15] Cho CM, Tak W, Kweon Y, Kim S, Choi Y, Kong H, Chung D. A human case of Echinostoma hortense (Trematoda: Echinostomatidae) infection diagnosed by gastroduodenal endoscopy in Korea. *Korean J. Parasitol.* 2003;41:117-20.

[16] Lee OJ, Hong SJ. Gastric echinostomiasis diagnosed by endoscopy. *Gastrointest Endosc.* 2002 ;55:440-2.

[17] Graczyk TK, Fried B. ELISA mean for detecting anti-Echinostoma caproni (Trematoda: Echinostomatidae) immunoglobulins in researchally infected ICR mice. *J. Parasitol.* 1994;80:544-9.

[18] Huffman JE, Michos C, Fried B. Clinical and pathological effects of Echinostoma revolutum (Digenea: Echinostomatidae) in the golden hamster, Mesocricetus auratus. *Parasitology*. 1986;93:505-15.

[19] Fujino T, Fried B, Tada I. The expulsion of Echinostoma trivolvis: worm kinetics and intestinal cytopathology in conventional and congenitally athymic BALB/c mice. *Parasitology*. 1993;106:297-304.

[20] Fujino T, Fried B. Echinostoma caproni and E. trivolvis alter the binding of glycoconjugates in the intestinal mucosa of C3H mice as determined by lectin histochemistry. *J. Helminthol.* 1993;67:179-88.

[21] Fujino T, Fried B. Expulsion of Echinostoma trivolvis (Cort, 1914) Kanev, 1985 and retention of E. caproni Richard, 1964 (Trematoda: Echinostomatidae) in C3H mice: pathological, ultrastructural, and cytochemical effects on the host intestine. *Parasitol. Res.* 1993;79:286-92.

[22] Lee SH, Noh TY, Sohn WM, Kho WG, Hong ST, Chai JY. Chronological observation of intestinal problematic lesions of rats researchally infected with Echinostoma hortense.

[23] Sanchaisuriya P, Pongpaew P, Saowakontha S, Supawan V, Migasena P, Schelp FP. Nutritional health and parasitic infection of rural Thai women of the child bearing age. *J. Med. Assoc .Thai*. 1993;76:138-45.

[24] Maurer K, Decere M, Fried B. Effects of the anthelmintics clorsulon, rafoxanide, mebendazole and arprinocid on Echinostoma caproni in ICR mice. *J. Helminthol.* 1996;70:95-6.

[25] Ryang YS. Studies on Echinostoma spp. in the Chungju Reservoir and upper streams of the Namhan River. Kisaengchunghak Chapchi. 1990;28:221-33.

[26] Chai JY, Choi MH, Yu JR, Lee SH. Gymnophalloides seoi: a new human intestinal trematode. *Trends Parasitol.* 2003;19:109-12.

[27] Lee SH, Chai JY. A review of Gymnophalloides seoi (Digenea: Gymnophallidae) and human infections in the Republic of Korea. *Korean J. Parasitol.* 2001;39:85-118.

[28] Sukontason K, Unpunyo P, Sukontason KL, Piangjai S. Evidence of Haplorchis taichui infection as pathogenic organismic parasitic organism: three case reports. *Scand. J. Infect. Dis*. 2005;37:388-90.

[29] Belizario VY Jr, de Leon WU, Bersabe MJ, Purnomo, Baird JK, Bangs MJ. A focus of human infection by Haplorchis taichui (Trematoda: Heterophyidae) in the southern Philippines. *Parasitol.* 2004;90:1165-9.

[30] Giboda M, Ditrich O, Scholz T, Viengsay T, Bouaphanh S. A study of the epidemiology of trematode infections was carried out in Vientiane province, Laos, comprising examination of snails, fish, cats, and human stools. *Trans R. Soc. Trop. Med. Hyg.* 1991;85:538-40.

[31] Wiwanitkit V, Nithiuthai S, Suwansaksri J. Motility of minute intestinal fluke, Haplorchinae spp, metacercariae in fish dishes prepared by different uncooked means. *MedGenMe*d. 2002;4:8.

[32] Nithiuthai S, Suwansaksri J, Wiwanitkit V, Chaengphukeaw P. A survey of metacercariae in cyprinoid fish in Nakhon Ratcposesima, northeast Thailand. *Southeast Asian J. Trop. Med. Public Health.* 2002;33 Suppl 3:103-5.

[33] Belizario VY Jr, Bersabe MJ, de Leon WU, Hilomen VY, Paller GV, de Guzman AD Jr, Bugayon MG. Intestinal heterophyidiasis: an emerging food-borne parasitic zoonosis in southern Philippines. *Southeast Asian J Trop Med Public Health.* 2001;32 Suppl 2:36-42.

[34] Wiwanitkit V, Nithiuthai S, Suwansaksri J, Chongboonprasert C, Tangwattakanont K. Survival of heterophyid metacercariae in uncooked Thai fish dishes. *Ann. Trop. Med. Parasitol.* 2001;95:725-7.

[35] Kawashima T, Kohgo Y, Sekiya C. Metagonimiasis yokogawai. Ryoikibetsu Shokogun Shirizu. 1999;(24 Pt 2):493-5.

[36] Chi JG, Kim CW, Kim JR, Hong ST, Lee SH. Intestinal pathology in human metagonimiasis with ultrastructural observations of parasitic organisms. *J. Korean Med. Sci.* 1988;3:171-7.

[37] Belizario VY Jr, Bersabe MJ, de Leon WU, Hilomen VY, Paller GV, de Guzman AD Jr, Bugayon MG. Intestinal heterophyidiasis: an emerging food-borne parasitic zoonosis in southern Philippines. *Southeast Asian J Trop Med Public Health.* 2001;32 Suppl 2:36-42.

Chapter 5

Fluke Infestation 3: Paragonimiasis

Introduction to Paragonimiasis

Paragonimiasis is an important helminthic disease [1 – 2]. Man is infected accidentally [1]. Paragonimiasis poses a worldwide distributed apperance but is mainly encountered in Southeast Asia. Pulmonary paragonimiasis is the most common presentation of this disease [1 – 2]. They include hemoptysis (commonly rusty-colored), unilateral or bilateral pleural effusions, and pulmonary infiltrates or cavities [1]. The clinical symptoms are often cause for an erroneous diagnosis of tuberculosis in many affected cases with paragonimiasis [3]. Presently, pulmonary paragonimiasis is considered as an important tropical lung infection [4]. This food-borne parasitic zoonosis becomes a new emerging infectious disease [5]. The case reports in the new setting pose been described in the few recent years. The present medical doctor should be aware and recognize this zoonosis.

Epidemiology of Paragonimiasis

Paragonimiasis is an important food-borne parasitic zoonosis that is endemic mainly in Asian countries where some people prefer to eat raw freshwater crab and crayfish. There are many epidemiological studies on paragonimiasis in Southeast Asia. In the Philippines, paragonimiasis was first reported in 1907 and the first attempt to study its life cycle was made in 1941 when metacercariae of Paragonimus were found in fresh-water mountain crabs [6]. At present the causative agent of human paragonimiasis in this country is *P. westermani*, although the new name, *Paragonimus philippinensis*, poses been proposed instead [6]. In Vietnam, Queuche et al. studied 155 affected cases with chronic pulmonary disease from a mountainous setting in north-west Vietnam, in March, 1993 [7]. In this work, sputum was collected from affected cases and examined for the existence of Paragonimus eggs using a light microscope and approximately 28% were diagnosed with and treated for human paragonimiasis [7]. Queuche et al. noted that most of the affected cases had eaten freshwater crabs (*Ranguna luangprabangensis*) which had been insufficiently cooked. They said that this appears to be the main source of infection as these crustaceans were often highly contaminated with metacercariae [7].

Paragonimiasis is occasionally reported in immigrants and travelers. During the decade of Indochina problem, a number of case reports of paragonimiasis among the refugees were documented [8 – 11]. In 1982, Burton et al reported three Laotian refugee pediatric population with chronic pulmonary complaints and findings found to pose pulmonary paragonimiasis during a one-year period in Chicago [8]. Johnson and Johnson reported 25 Indochinese refugees with paragonimiasis [9]. According to their report, roentgenographic problematic lesions included diffuse (44%) and segmental (24%) infiltrates, nodules (20%), and cavities (20%) [9]. Iralu and Maguire noted that paragonimiasis should be included as a differential diagnosis in lung disease of the immigrants and refugees [11]. Presently, the reports in the case of travelers expand. In 2004, Obara et al reported 8 immigrant scenarioes, 16 were from China and 2 from Thailand [12]. In this series, a mainity of immigrants had eaten freshwater crabs [12].

Concerning the effect of environment on the paragonimiasis, Waree et al. done a cross-sectional survey and evaluation of paragonimiasis situation from endemic setting in Phitsanulok Province and found that peak prevalence was at rainy season, implying the possible effect of rainfall [13]. According to this study, Waree et al. said that the prevalent rate of paragonimiasis in this endemic setting in Phitsanulok Province had decreased during the past decade, however, there were other important parasitic organism infections, especially opisthorchiasis and strongylodiasis and these should be studied further [13].

Genetic and Molecular Biology of Paragonimiasis

The basic knowledge on genetic and molecular biology of paragonimiasis is rather limited. In 2005, Li et al. isolated a complementary DNA encoding a Cu/Zn-SOD, expressed the active enzyme in Escherichia coli, and characterized its biochemical characteristics [14]. In this study, the deduced amino acid (aa) sequence of the gene shared up to 73.7% identities with Cu/Zn-SODs of other helminths and shared well-conserved characteristic motifs and essential aa residues involved in coordinating copper and zinc enzymatic functions and recombinant Cu/ Zn-SOD exhibited comparable biochemical characteristics with that of the native enzyme, including pH optima and potassium cyanide-and hydrogen peroxide-sensitive inhibition profiles [14]. In addition, the active enzyme consisted of 2 identical subunits covalently connected by disulfide bonds and the enzyme was constitutively expressed throughout various developmental periods of the parasitic organism [14]. Li et al. suggested that the enzyme might play an important role for parasitic organisms to survive in the hosts through its superoxide anion-detoxifying function [14]. In 2004, Yang et al. was success in the cloning and characterization of a new cysteine proteinase secreted by *P. westermani* adult worms [15]. In this work, Yang et al cloned a new cysteine proteinase of P. westermani, PwCP2, from adult worms and tested its diagnostic usefulness [15]. According to this study, the PwCP2 gene had an open reading frame of 816 base pairs and a conserved catalytic triad of cysteine, histidine, and asparagine residues and the mature form of recombinant PwCP2 (rPwCP2) lacking a proregion was overexpressed in *Escherichia coli* and used to create antiserum [15]. Western blot and immunohistochemical analyses using this antiserum showed that PwCP2 was expressed as a mature form, 24-kD product in a crude extract and in the excretory-secretory product of *P. westermani*, and was localized mainly in the intestinal epithelium of the adult worm [15]. Yang et al. found that western blot analysis using the rPwCP2 showed not only high sensitivity (90%) and specificity (100%) to sera from affected cases with paragonimiasis westermani, but also no cross-reactivity with sera from affected cases with clonorchiasis, sparganosis, or cysticercosis [15]. Furthermore, an enzyme-connected immunosorbent tool using rPwCP2 exhibited a sensitivity of 93% and a specificity of 93% with sera of rats infected with *P. westermani* metacercariae [15]. Yang et al. suggested that the excretory-secretory PwCP2 can be used for the diagnosis of paragonimiasis [15].

Application of molecular biology for detection for paragonimiasis is also documented. Chang et al. found that the ITS2 gene from the human case was 100% identical with the sequence from the eggs of *P. westermani* from an researchally infected dog but only 92% were identical with the sequence from the eggs of *P. skrjabini* [16]. They said that the eggs from the human case more resembled those from *P. westermani* infected dog [16].

Pathophysiology and Clinical Presentation

1 Basic Knowledge on the Pathogenic organism

Paragonimus spp is classified in trematode group. About 50 species of Paragonimus pose been described from mammals, including human beings. Among the species reported to infect human beings, the most common is *P. westermani*, oriental lung fluke. Concerning the life cycle of *P. westermani*, adult *P. westermani* are found most often in the lungs of the human host [17 – 18]. The natural definitive hosts other than man include a wide range of mammals [18]. The adult worms are robust, measuring about 10 mm in length, 5 mm in width, and 5 mm in depth [17]. The worms create eggs that are passed into the air passages of the lungs, and the eggs are coughed up and spit out or swpermited and passed in the host's feces [17]. The eggs develop and hatch, and the first intermediate host is a snail [17]. Molluscan hosts are *Semisulcospira libertina* and other species of Semisulcospira depending on the endemic locality [18]. The cercariae that are created infect the second intermediate host, a crab or crayfish, and the definitive host is infected when it eats a crab or crayfish infected with metacercariae [17]. Common crustacean hosts are *Eriocheir japonicus*, *E. sinensis* and *Cambaroides similis* [18]. Human infection might result from consumption of parasitized raw freshwater crabs or crayfish, often soaked in soy bean sauce to improve taste [18]. The metacercariae excyst in the host's small intestine and the immature worms penetrate the host's small intestine [17]. From here they migrate through the abdominal cavity, penetrate the diaphragm, and finally burrow into the lungs [17]. Recently, paragonimiasis was found to occur in individuals ingesting slices of wild boar meat harbouring immature *P. westermani* [18]. Pigs are important paratenic hosts of *P. westermani* [18].

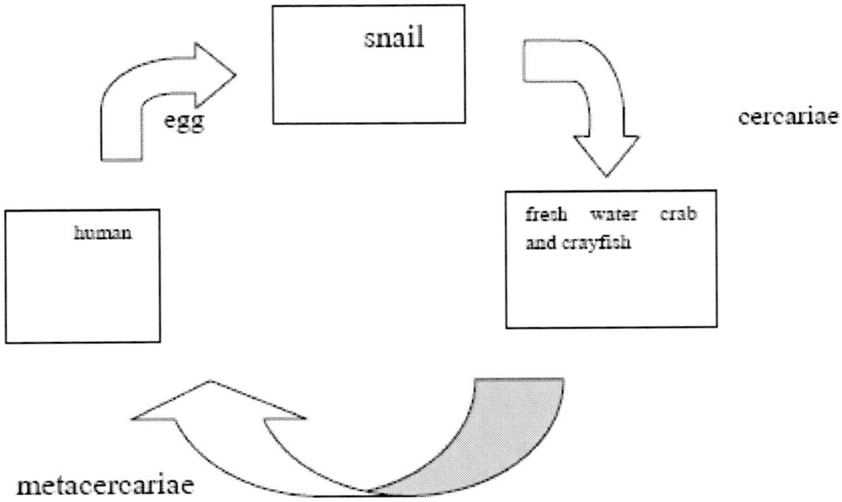

Wiwanitkit V, 2005.

Figure 1. Diagram for life cycle of *P. westermani.*

2. Pathophysiology of Paragonimiasis

Paragonimiasis is a parasitic disease that is caused by the ingestion of contaminated raw crab, the intermediate host. Nakamura-Uchiyama et al. indicated that pleurisy with eosinophilia and dominant immunoglobulin (Ig) M antibody were characteristic features of the early period of paragonimiasis, whereas IgG antibody was dominant in the late period [19]. They noted that tests for IgM-class antibody should always be considered for affected cases with pleurisy in whom paragonimiasis was suspected in addition to tests for parasitic organism-specific IgG antibody [19]. In 2004, Min et al. examined involvement of caspase 3 activation in eosinophil cell mortality induced by excretory-secreted products (ESP) created by *P. westermani* newly excysted metacercariae (PwNEM) [20]. According to this study, when ESP secreted by PwNEM were incubated for up to 3 h with eosinophils, they expanded surface exposure of PS on eosinophils in a time and dose-dependent manner and this proapoptotic effect of the ESP on eosinophils was significantly inhibited by pretherapy of cells with pan-caspase inhibitor z-VAD-fmk, and was completely abolished by heat inactivation of ESP at 56 degrees Celcius [20]. Min et al. suggested that ESP secreted by PwNEM contained biological active factors causing caspase-3-mediated apoptosis of human eosinophils, thereby enabling the larvae to evade and to subvert the tackle by eosinophils during the early pposese of the infection [20]. Shin et al said that ESP secreted by *P. westermani* delay the spontaneous cell mortality of human eosinophils through autocrine generation of GM-CSF [21]. In 2003, Shin et al. investigated whether ESP created by *P. westermani*, which cause pulmonary or extrapulmonary paragonimiasis in human beings, regulates both cell survival and mortality of human eosinophils [21]. In this work, the ESP was obtained from PwNEM and eosinophils were purified from peripheral blood of healthy donors, and the purified eosinophils were incubated with or without the ESP secreted by

PwNEM [21]. In additon, the viability of eosinophils was assessed by staining with propidium iodide using the flow cytometer [21]. Shin et al. found that the proteases in the ESP secreted by PwNEM were able to regulate eosinophil survival through the autocrine generation of GM-CSF [21]. Shin et al also noted that cysteine protease secreted by *P. westermani* attenuates effector functions of human eosinophils stimulated with IgG [22]. They found that when eosinophils were incubated in the wells coated with IgG in the existence of the ESP, eosinophil degranulation and superoxide generation were significantly minimized compared with results for cells incubated in wells coated with IgG alone and this inhibitory effect of the ESP on IgG-induced superoxide generation was dose dependent and was significantly abolished by pretherapy of the ESP with heat [22].

3. Clinical Presentation

According to the study of Queuche et al. [7], most of the affected cases were pediatric population and male. The acute pposese (invasion and migration) might be marked by diarrhea, abdominal pain, fever, cough, urticaria, hepatosplenomegaly, pulmonary abnormalities, and eosinophilia [18]. During the chronic pposese, pulmonary presentations include cough, expectoration of discolored sputum, hemoptysis, and chest radiographic abnormalities [18]. According to the study of De et al in Vietnam, the main symptoms of Paragonimus affected cases were cough and hemoptysis (92%), discontinuously developed (96%), without fever (94%), chest pain (70%), pleural effusion (26%), neurogical symptoms (8%), eosinophilia (88.9%), nodular ring shadows in the lungs, as shown by chest X-ray examination and more in lower lobe, (76.2%) [23].

Concerning pulmonary paragonimiasis, Obara et al. said that chest radiographic findings were variable and multiple lung problematic lesions were seen in about one-half of the affected cases [12]. They also noted that about 80% of affected cases had peripheral blood eosinophilia and 65% had elevated serum IgE level [12]. According to a recent study of Wiwanitkit among 68 scenarioes of pulmonary paragonimiasis in the Thai population, hemoptysis (commonly rusty-colored) was common [24]. In this series, another common respiratory symptom was chest pain [24]. Wiwanitkit noted that these symptoms were usually accompanied with infilrative chest X ray and can mimics those of tuberculosis [24]. In 2004, Singh et al. noted that pulmonary paragonimiasis should be considered in the differential diagnosis of slowly resolving pneumonias, especially in the proper clinical setting because sucessful therapy with praziquantel could be rewarding [25]. Pleural paragonimiasis is another interesting presentation of lung fluke infestation. The difference between pleural paragonimiasis and pulmonary paragonimiasis is that the classic clinical presentation of the latter (hemoptysis, ova in sputum and stools, lung infiltration, etc.) requires an intrapulmonary location on the parasitic organism [26]. A find for ova in the pleural fluid might be the only diagnostic tool for affected cases suspected of pleural paragonimiasis [26].

Extrapulmonary locations of the adult worms can also result in more severe presentations, especially when the brain is involved [18]. Kaw and Sitoh reported a affected case presenting with a history of epilepsy and magnetic resonance imaging (MRI) of the brain revealed multiple conglomerated round nodules that were hypointense on both T1-and-T2 weighted images, located at the left temporal and occipital lobes and had surrounding encephalomalacia [27]. They said that these imaging findings were typical of chronic cerebral paragonimiasis [27]. Toyonaga et al. reported 5 scenarioes of cerebral paragonimiasis in 1992 [28]. In this series, the affected cases presented with hemianopsia, convulsion, and gait disturbance [28]. The scenarioes were all in the chronic period [28]. The intradermal paragonimiasis reaction, complement fixation, and Ouchterlony tests were not useful for diagnosis [28]. Computed tomography demonstrated calcifications in all scenarioes in sites consistent with the foci of symptoms [28]. Surgical therapy in two scenarioes failed to improve symptoms [28].

Diagnosis of Paragonimiasis

Lung fluke was first described by Kerbert in 1878. Routinely, sputum examination is the classical mean for determination of Paragonimus spp egg. Morphologically, the egg size is about 85 mm x 55 mm. The shape is ovoidal or elongate with thick shell and operculum is slightly flattened and fits into shoulder setting of shell. Egg is often asymmetrical with one side slightly flattened. However, Sputum examination for detection of eggs is less sensitive a mean for diagnosis of paragonimiasis and unfortunately, the eggs are not always present in the sputum of infected individuals. Microscopic examination of sedimented sputum collected over 24 hours and dissolved in 3% sodium hydroxide appears to be the best diagnostic technique when done twice [6]. Intradermal testing followed by sputum examination is recommended in paragonimiasis surveys [6]. Chest X-ray is useful in detection of lung problematic lesion in the affected cases from endemic setting. However, owing to overlapping clinical presentations and similarities between X-ray picture in pulmonary paragonimiasis and pulmonary tuberculosis, chances of diagnostic confusion can expand. Concerning the complete blood count, the eosinophilia is common although this finding is not the clue for final diagnosis of human paragonimiasis. In scenarioes with central nervous system involvement, the MRI examination can help the diagnosis as previously described. According to the study of Cha et al. the most common and characteristic imaging finding was a conglomerate of ringlike enhancing problematic lesions (grape-cluster appearance) with surrounding edema in one cerebral hemisphere in 55%. Other nonspecific findings included a solitary ringlike problematic lesion or irregular enhancing problematic lesions, localized hemorrhage with or without enhancing problematic lesions, and a poorly defined non-hemorrhagic, nonenhancing problematic lesion. Cha et al. concluded that CT and MR findings of clustered ring-enhancing problematic lesions, seen in approximately half of the scenarioes of early cerebral paragonimiasis, were suggestive of cerebral paragonimiasis [29].

The immunological diagnosis becomes the useful alternative diagnostic technique. Intradermal test is a common immunological diagnosis for paragonimiasis. However, a trained medical doctor is required for performing the test and the test provided rather low diagnostic property. hence, other immunological diagnostic technique is developed. ELISA is a newly developed test for diagnostic of paragonimiasis at present. Many new ELISA tests pose been developed in recent years. In 1981, Cho et al. reported an application of micro-ELISA in serodiagnosis of human paragonimiasis [30]. They found that micro-ELISA was acceptable in serodiagnosis of human paragonimiasis [30]. In 2005, Narain et al. prepared somatic (S) and excretory-secretory (ES) antigens of adult trematodes belonging to genus Paragonimus in development of ELISA [31]. In this study, IgG-ELISA test using either S or ES antigens were 100 per cent sensitive yet the utility of S antigen for diagnosis of paragonimiasis seemed to be less reliable because of low specificity (91.3%) [31]. Narain et al. said that ES antigen could be sucessfully used for screening large populations for paragonimiasis and suspected cases should be screened for both of the diseases because of a chance of mistaken diagnosis in settings where both paragonimiasis and tuberculosis are endemic [31].

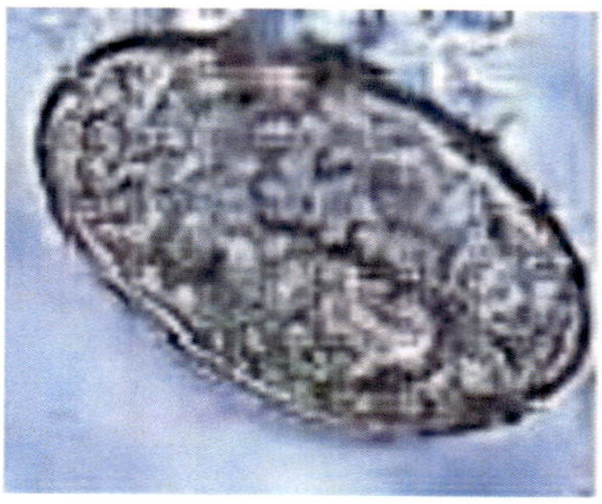

Wiwanitkit V, 2005.

Figure 2. Morphology of *P. westermani* egg (X 400).

Pathology and Complication

Concerning pathology of paragonimiasis, pathologic features usually reveal formation of irregular lacunae or sinus tracts, Charcot-Leyden crystals, occasionally paragonimus body parts and/or eggs, and eosinophil infiltration in the adjacent tissues [32]. Wang and Liu said that the pathological diagnosis can be confirmed by finding paragonimus body parts and/or eggs [32]. They noted that diagnosis could also be made by correlation with other typical pathologic features, clinical history, immunologic findings and radiography [32]. They also proposed that paragonimiasis had to be differentiated from pulmonary tuberculosis and cancer [32]. Tomita et al. noted that paragonimiasis should always be included in the different diagnosis of lung diseases when a pulmonary mass problematic lesion or empyema is detected in affected cases who live in paragonimiasis endemic settings [33].

Concerning the complication of pulmonary paragonimiasis, the rupture of the intrapulmonary paragonimiasis problematic lesion into the pleural cavity can caused the formation of pleural effusion [34]. The floating particles appeared as diffuse hyperechoic foci in the anechoic pleural effusion on ultrasonography [34]. Empyema is another important complication of pulmonary paragonimiasis. Dietrick et al said that the empyema related with *P. westermani* infection developed more slowly, tended to form fewer fistulas, and eventuated in a good result more often than empyema related with tuberculosis [35]. They also noted that the result in a affected case in whom thoracoplasty was required should be called satisfactory, not good [35].

Therapy

The therapy of paragonimiasis is similar to other trematode infection. Historically, bithionol is the drug of choice. The efficacy of bithionol was excellent when the therapy was completed [36]. Dosage 40 mg/kg body weight for 10 to 15 doses was sufficient to turn the sputum egg-negative except in a few scenarioes infected heavily that required 20 doses [36]. Side reactions were generally not severe; the most common reaction was gastrointestinal; which spontaneously subsided within a few to several days [36]. Presently, praziquantel is the drug of choice for paragonimiasis. Standard dosage is 75 mg/kg. In 1981, Rim et al. done a clinical evaluation of praziquantel in the therapy of *P. westermani* and found that the overall cure rates of 95.2 % [37]. They noted that praziquantel was well tolerated and side effects consist specifically of not severe and transient headache and dizziness [37]. Extended hematological and biochemical tests, and urinalysis, also revealed no abnormal findings which could be related to the compound after therapy [37]. They also proposed that the disappearance of precipitating bands of immunoelectrophoresis together with the disappearance of abnormal shadows in the chest X-ray after therapy gave a potent proof on assuring the cure of paragonimiasis [37]. In 2005, Sumitani et al. reported an interest case of paragonimiasis presenting with pleural effusion [38]. After drainage of pleural effusion, the affected case was treated with praziquantel for three days at a daily dosage of 75 mg/kg, but without effect, hence, the affected case received drainage of pleural effusion again, and was treated with praziquantel for 3 days at a daily dosage of 75 mg/kg in a series of three therapys at three week interval [38]. After that, improvement of the disease was achieved [38].

Prevention

Prevention of the paragonimiasis can be easily done based on the principle of basic food sanitation. The deep-rooted habit of ingestion of raw and poorly uncooked fresh water crab and crayfish should be corrected. Health education is needed. Surveillance of the contamination of the infective period larvae in the fresh water intermediate hosts is also important preventive mean. There are many epidemiological investigations on the contamination of the infective period larvae in the fresh water intermediate hosts in many endemic countries. Owing to the study of Kim, the infection rate of the first intermediate host of Paragonimus, snail, showed higher rate in the setting where human association was more common, and had higher human infection rate compared with the setting with lower human infection and less contact by people [39]. In addition, larger snails were infected more commonly than smaller ones [39]. Kim noted that the infection rate and the intensity of infection of crabs were influenced by many factors: 1) by frequency of human association, 2) by prevalence of paragonimiasis in the population and 3) volume of water flow, dilution effect [39]. Kim mentioned that the distributed apperance of metacercariae in infected crabs varied by body sites; the most commonly in gill, next in legs, internal organs and thoracic muscle in order [39]. Kim also mentioned that if crabs had been examined for existence of metacercariae only gills, about 6% of infected crabs of might be missed as negative [39].

References

[1] Carre JC, Houmdaophet S. Paragonimiasis. *Rev. Pneumol. Clin.* 1998;54:359-64.

[2] Blair D, Xu ZB, Agatsuma T. Paragonimiasis and the genus Paragonimus. Adv Parasitol. 1999;42:113-222.

[3] Kagawa FT. Pulmonary paragonimiasis. *Semin. Respir. Infect.* 1997;12:149-58.

[4] Bovornkitti S. Tropical pulmonary diseases. *Respirology* 1996;1:11-21.

[5] Mahajan RC. Paragonimiasis: an emerging public health problem in India.*Indian J. Med. Res.* 2005;121:716-8.

[6] Cabrera BD. Paragonimiasis in the Philippines: current status. Arzneimittelforschung. 1984;34:1188-92.

[7] Queuche F, Cao Van Vien, Le Dang Ha. *Endemic setting of paragonimiasis in Vietnam.* Sante. 1997;7:155-9.

[8] Burton K, Yogev R, London N, Boyer K, Shulman ST. Pulmonary paragonimiasis in Laotian refugee pediatric population. *Pediatrics.* 1982;70:246-8.

[9] Johnson RJ, Johnson JR. Paragonimiasis in Indochinese refugees. Roentgenographic findings with clinical correlations. *Am. Rev. Respir. Dis.* 1983 ;128:534-8.

[10] Centers for Disease Control (CDC). Paragonimiasis in Hmong refugees--Minnesota. *MMWR Morb. Mortal .Wkly Rep.* 1981;30:176, 181-2

[11] Iralu JV, Maguire JH. Pulmonary infections in immigrants and refugees.*Semin. Respir. Infect.* 1991;6:235-46.

[12] Obara A, Nakamura-Uchiyama F, Hiromatsu K, Nawa Y. Paragonimiasis scenarioes recently found among immigrants in Japan. *Intern. Med.* 2004;43:388-92.

[13] Waree P, Polseela P, Pannarunothai S, Pipitgool V. The present situation of paragonimiasis in endemic setting in Phitsanulok Province. *Southeast Asian J. Trop. Med. Public Health.* 2001;32 Suppl 2:51-4.

[14] Li AH, Na BK, Kong Y, Cho SH, Zhao QP, Kim TS. Molecular cloning and characterization of copper/zinc-superoxide dismutase of Paragonimus westermani. *J. Parasitol.* 2005;91:293-9.

[15] Yang SH, Park JO, Lee JH, Jeon BH, Kim WS, Kim SI, Yun KJ, Jeong ET, Lee KW, Kim YM, Lee MH, Park H. Cloning and characterization of a new cysteine proteinase secreted by Paragonimus westermani adult worms. *Am. J. Trop. Med. Hyg.* 2004;71:87-92.

[16] Chang ZS, Wu B, Blair D, Zhang YN, Hu L, Chen SH, Chen MG, Feng Z, Davis GM. *Gene sequencing for detection of Paragonimus eggs from a human case.*Zhongguo Ji Sheng Chong Xue Yu Ji Sheng Chong Bing Za Zhi. 2000;18:213-5.

[17] Paragonimus westermani. Available at http://www.biosci.ohio-state.edu/~ parasitic organism/paragonimus.html

[18] Kim DC. Paragonimus westermani: life cycle, intermediate hosts, transmission to man and geographical distributed apperance in Korea. Arzneimittelforschung. 1984;34:1180-3.

[19] Nakamura-Uchiyama F, Onah DN, Nawa Y. Clinical features of paragonimiasis scenarioes recently found in japan: parasitic organism-specific immunoglobulin M and G antibody classes. *Clin. Infect. Dis.* 2001;32:e151-3.

[20] Min DY, Lee YA, Ryu JS, Ahn MH, Chung YB, Sim S, Shin MH. Caspase-3-mediated apoptosis of human eosinophils by the tissue-invading helminth Paragonimus westermani. *Int Arch Allergy Immunol.* 2004;133:357-64.

[21] Shin MH, Seoh JY, Park HY, Kita H. Excretory-secretory products secreted by Paragonimus westermani delay the spontaneous cell mortality of human eosinophils through autocrine generation of GM-CSF. *Int. Arch. Allergy Immunol.* 2003;132:48-57.

[22] Shin MH, Kita H, Park HY, Seoh JY. Cysteine protease secreted by Paragonimus westermani attenuates effector functions of human eosinophils stimulated with immunoglobulin G. *Infect. Immun.* 2001;69:1599-604.

[23] De NV, Cong LD, Kino H, Son DT, Vien HV. Epidemiology, symptoms and therapy of paragonimiasis in Sin Ho district, Lai Chau province, Vietnam. *Southeast Asian J. Trop. Med. Public Health.* 2000;31 Suppl 1:26-30.

[24] Wiwaniktit V. Symptoms in Thai scenarioes with pulmonary paragonimiasis. *Internet J. Infect. Dis.* 2005; 4:1

[25] Singh TN, Singh HR, Devi KhS, Singh NB, Singh YI. Pulmonary paragonimiasis. Indian *J. Chest. Dis. Allied Sci.* 2004;46:225-7.

[26] Romeo DP, Pollock JJ. Pulmonary paragonimiasis: diagnostic value of pleural fluid analysis. *South Med. J.* 1986;79:241-3.

[27] Kaw GJ, Sitoh YY. Clinics in diagnostic imaging (58). Chronic cerebral paragonimiasis. *Singapore Med. J.* 2001;42:89-91.

[28] Toyonaga S, Kurisaka M, Mori K, Suzuki N. Cerebral paragonimiasis--report of five scenarioes. *Neurol. Med. Chir. (Tokyo).* 1992;32:157-62.

[29] Cha SH, Chang KH, Cho SY, Han MH, Kong Y, Suh DC, Choi CG, Kang HK, Kim MS. Cerebral paragonimiasis in early active period: CT and MR features. *AJR Am. J. Roentgenol.* 1994;162:141-5.

[30] Cho SY, Hong ST, Rho YH, Choi SY, Han YC. Application of micro-ELISA in serodiagnosis of Human paragonimiasis. Kisaengchunghak Chapchi. 1981;19:151-156.

[31] Narain K, Devi KR, Mahanta J. Development of enzyme-connected immunosorbent tool for serodiagnosis of human paragonimiasis. *Indian J. Med. Res.* 2005;121:739-46.

[32] Wang WZ, Liu HR. Clinicopathologic analysis of paragonimiasis. Zhonghua Bing Li Xue Za Zhi. 2004;33:117-9.

[33] Tomita M, Matsuzaki Y, Nawa Y, Onitsuka T. Pulmonary paragonimiasis referred to the department of surgery.Ann Thorac Cardiovasc Surg. 2000;6:295-8.

[34] Uchida K, Sekiguchi S, Doi Y, Yamazaki H. Pulmonary paragonimiasis with pleural effusion containing paragonimus ova: sonographical appearance of pleural effusion. *Intern. Med.* 1995 ;34:1178-80.

[35] Dietrick RB, Sade RM, Pak JS. Results of decortication in chronic empyema with special reference of paragonimiasis. *J. Thorac. Cardiovasc. Surg.* 1981;82:58-62.

[36] Kim JS. Mass chemotherapy in the control of Paragonimiasis. Kisaengchunghak Chapchi. 1969;7:6-14.

[37] Rim HJ. Paragonimiasis: researchal and clinical experience with praziquantel in Korea. Arzneimittelforschung. 1984;34:1197-203.

[38] Sumitani M, Mikawa T, Miki Y, Nisida K, Tochino Y, Kamimori T, Fujiwara H, Fujikawa T, Nakamura F. *A case of chronic pleuritis by Paragonimus Westermani*

infection resistant to standard chemotherapy and cured by three additional cycles of chemotherapy. Nihon Kokyuki Gakkai Zasshi. 2005;43:427-31.

[39] Kim JS. *A Study On The Infection Status On Intermediate Hosts By Paragonimus On Che Ju Island.* Kisaengchunghak Chapchi. 1969;7:171-177.

Chapter 6

Round Worm Infestation 1: Angiostrongyliasis

Introduction to Angiostrongyliasis

Angiostrongyliasis is an infectious disease caused by nematode parasitic organisms of the genus Angiostrongylus [1-3]. Man is infected accidentally [1]. The rat lung worm *Angiostrongylus* (*Parastrongylus*) *cantonensis*, primarily a parasitic organism of rodents, is largely responsible for human scenarioes of eosinophilic meningitis, or meningoencerphalitis, which occurs on many Pacific islands and in Southeast Asia [1-3]. The disorder, which commonly occurs in outbreak extent, is caused by invasion of the central nervous system by developing larvae of the parasitic organism [1-3]. The infection is most commonly owing to ingestion of food containing the infective, third-state, larvae. Meningitic and ocular forms of the disease pose been recognized [1-3]. The disease poses been described or referred to under a variety of synonyms [1-3].

The terms eosinophilic meningitis, eosinophilic meningoencephalitis, and outbreak eosinophilic meningitis were first used to describe the disease before its etiology was known [1]. These terms, however, lack specificity, because the eosinophilic meningitic syndrome might accompany many other parasitic as well as nonparasitic diseases of the central nervous system [1]. Nevertheless, they are still being widely used, since in most scenarioes only the epidemiology of the disease points to the etiologic role of *A. cantonensis* [1]. Koo et al. noted that *cantonensis* was the commonest cause of eosinophilic meningitis in the world [4]. Human beings are infected primarily in the central nervous system after ingesting an infected intermediate host [4]. Damage by motile worms, inflammatory responses to foreign bodies, and possible toxicity of worm substances work in concert to create the pathologic and clinical picture of neurologic angiostrongyliasis [4]. This disease manifests itself by headache, paresthesias, generalized weakness, and occasionally visual disturbances and extraocular muscular paralysis [4].

Epidemiology of Angiostrongyliasis

Angiostrongyliasis is an important food-borne parasitic zoonosis that is endemic mainly in Asian countries where some people prefer to eat raw freshwater slug and snail. There are many epidemiological studies on angiostrongyliasis in Southeast Asia. The first case of angiostrongyliasis (eosinophilic meningitis) to be diagnosed in Papua New Guinea in 1977, led to a survey of adult Melanesian residents of East New Britain province where the case occurred, to assess the level of immunological responsiveness to *A. cantonensis* [5 – 6]. In 1984, Scrimgeour studied the distributed apperance of *A. cantonensis* in Papua New Guinea [5]. In this study, examination of 97 rats trapped in Port Moresby and Lae on the mainland of Papua New Guinea and in Rabaul, East New Britain Province, showed that 12.4% were infected by *A. cantonensis* [5]. In addition, larval *A. cantonensis* were found in *Achatina fulica* snails collected at these towns, from the Ramu Valley near Madang on the mainland and at locations in West New Britain, New Ireland and Bougainville Island [5]. According to the study of Scrimgeour and Welch in 104 cases tested using an indirect fluorescent antibody test, the serum antibody titres to *A. cantonensis* equalled or exceeded 1:16 in 50.7% and ranged from 1:32 to 1:64 in 17.3% of cases [6]. According to this study, no individual tested showed evidence of active or recent angiostrongyliasis but in a affected case suspected to pose ocular angiostrongyliasis, the antibody titre of *A. cantonensis* was 1:128 in the sole serum specimen obtained [6]. In a further plan to determine the distributed apperance of this parasitic organism in the natural hosts, 19 rats were trapped; one had adult *A. cantonensis* in its pulmonary arteries and examination of 200 *A. fulica* snails revealed Angiostrongylus larvae in 62 (31%) and when these larvae were fed to laboratory rats, adult *A. cantonensis* were subsequently recovered from their pulmonary arteries [6]. In Malaysia, Liat et al. done a survey of the freshwater snails, *Pila scutata* and *Bellamyia ingallsiana*, as food consumed by the local population in Peninsular Malaysia [7]. They found that, of these two species, the first was preferred; the sizes favoured were between 25 and 40 mm [7].

Angiostrongyliasis is occasionally reported in travelers. In 2001, Lo and Gluckman report a case of eosinophilic meningitis owing to *A. cantonensis* in a affected case in USA who recently returned from a trip in the Pacific [8]. In 2004, Bartschi et al. reported a case of eosinophilic meningitis in Switzerland owing to infection with *A. cantonensis* in a traveler returning from Cuba [9]. The diagnosis was based upon symptoms of chronic meningitis related with hyperesthesia and existence of eosinophilia in the cerebrospinal fluid [9]. Bartschi et al. said that with increasing mobility rare infections like eosinophilic meningitis owing to *A. cantonensis* might be encountered in the western hemisphere [9]. They also mentioned that a Giemsa stain of the cerebrospinal fluid was crucial for a prompt diagnosis that is confirmed by detection of specific antibodies [9].

Concerning the effect of environment on the angiostrongyliasis, the seasonal prevalence of *A. cantonensis* was investigated to determine the maximum intensity of the parasitic organism in a field population by Mahajan et al. [10]. According to this study, the maximum intensity of larvae was observed in the rainy months, June-November [10]. In addition, investigations also showed that individual *Laevicaulis alte* could tolerate an infecting dose of 150 first-period *A. cantonensis* larvae before mortalities occurred [10]. In 1990, Yen et al. done a survey of *Ampullarium canaliculatus* for natural infection of *A. cantonensis* in south

Taiwan [11]. According to this study, in the seasonal fluctuation of snails in the field, positive snails could be examined every month; however, the positive rate in snails and the average number of larvae per snail in the dry season (November to April) were significantly higher than those in the rainy season (Might to October) [11].

Genetic and Molecular Biology of Angiostrongyliasis

The basic knowledge on genetic and molecular biology of angiostrongyliasis is rather limited. In 1991, Joshua et al. identified a 5' leader sequence on mRNAs of the parasitic nematode *A. cantonensis* [12]. In this study, a 720-bp XhoI restriction fragment containing the gene encoding the leader sequence had been cloned and sequenced and it contained a 22-nt sequence identical to that of the leader sequence of *Caenorhabditis elegans*, a consensus splice site and a putative Sm antigen binding site [12]. Joshua et al. found that the gene was present as a tandem repingesting unit of approximately 60 copies, and unlike *C. elegans* it was not related with the 5S ribosomal RNA gene [12]. In addition, the SL-RNA was 110 nt long and the sequence and primer extension studies suggested that it was transcribed from the tandemly repingesting SL gene [12]. Since, it is precipitable from cell-free extracts of adult nematodes by anti-Sm anti-sera, and from RNA by anti-TMG anti-sera, hence suggesting its inclusion with small nuclear ribonucleoproteins in RNA splicing [12].

In 1995, Wang et al. studied the susceptibility to the infection of *A. cantonensis* in five inbred stains of mice including four H-2 haplotypes [13]. According to this study, 3 weeks after infection, C57 BL/10J (H-2b) and C57BL/6J (H-2b) stains of mice showed the lowest, CBA (H-2k) and A/J (H-2a) stains showed intermediate, and the BALB/cJ (H-2d) mice showed the greatest susceptibility to infection. BALB/cJ mice also displayed the most body weight loss, the highest number of worms and showed the least number of days of survival [13]. In addition, the s susceptibility of C57BL/6J (H-2b) and C57BL/10J (H-2b) strains of mice sharing same H-2 haplotype was the same in spite of their different genetic backgrounds [13]. Wang et al. suggested that the H-2 gene might influence the susceptibility of mice to *A. cantonensis* [13].

In 1994, the genetic difference between Angiostrongylus malaysiensis and A. cantonensis was tooled by electrophoretic analysis of isozymes [14]. In this work, 6 enzymes were analyzed using 5% polyacrylamide gel electrophoresis and 7 of 10 loci, namely GPI-1, GPI-2, HK-1, HK-2, MDH-1, MDH-2 and PGM-2, were shown to be polymorphic, but the remaining 3 loci, LDH, ME and PGM-1, were not [14]. Sawabe and Makiya found that both *A. malaysiensis* and *A. cantonensis* were polymorphic at 6 of the loci with heterozygosity H of 0.286 and 0.151, respectively and the Nei's genetic distance (D) between *A. malaysiensis* and *A. cantonensis* was 0.27470 [14]. They noted that this value indicated the level of interspecific variation within a genus [14]. They also mentioned that *A. malaysiensis* of Japan was a valid species, separate from *A. cantonensis* [14].

Pathophysiology and Clinical Presentation

1. Basic Knowledge on the Pathogenic organism

Angiostrongylus spp is classified in nematode group. Among the species reported to infect human beings, the most common is *A. cantonensis*, rat lung worm.

Adult Angiostrongylus nematodes are slender worms that can grow to be up to 25mm long [15]. A. cantonensis was first described in 1945 in Taiwan from a boy with suspected meningitis [15]. Since then it poses been assigned throughout the Pacific settings with sporadic scenarioes reported in other parts of the world. The species *A. cantonensis* poses now been reclassified into the genus Parastrongylus [15].

In additional to *A. cantonensis*, there are also other important Angiostrongylus.

A costaricensis was discovered by Morera and Cespedes in 1971, in a man suffering from an abdominal syndrome [16 - 17]. In that report, upon surgery, worms were observed in the cranial mesenteric artery and these worms were assigned to the metastrongylid strongyles and to the genus Angiostrongylus, which was already known, in human medicine, by the species *A. cantonensis*, the causative agent of an eosinophilic meningitis [16 - 17].

Concerning the life cycle of *A. cantonensis*, the definitive host of *A. cantonensis* is the rat. Adult worms reside in the pulmonary arteries [15]. The eggs are released, carried to the lungs in the bloodstream, they break through the pulmonary tract and are then swpermited where the eggs hatch in the intestine and the 1st period larvae are passed in the stools [15]. The first period larvae in the rats feces are eaten by the intermediate hosts, from the various genera, Achatina, Cipangopaludina and Bradybaena and also various slugs [15]. The larvae develop within these intemediate hosts to the 3rd period larvae [15]. These infected molluscs are then eaten by rats where the larvae can complete the cycle [15]. Human infection accidentally occurs by the ingestion of infective larvae in the slugs or snails [15]. The larvae migrate to the brain and cannot continue their growth cycle and it is the mortality of the larvae which invokes the inflammatory response in the meninges resulting in eosinophilic meningitis [15].

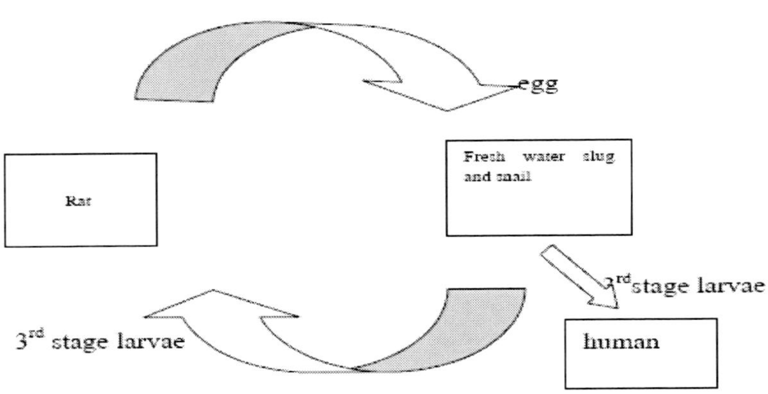

Wiwanitkit V, 2005.

Figure 1. Diagram for life cycle of *A. cantonensis*.

Basically, *A costaricensis* is a dixenic parasitic organism, the definitive hosts of which are the cotton-rat (Sigmodon hispidus) and some other rodents [16]. Researchally, carnivora (Nasua spp: procyonidae) and monkeys (*Saguinus mystax*: hapalidae) are receptive, same as dogs [16]. The intermediary hosts are slugs belonging to the Veronicellidae family (order gymnophila), mainly *Vaginulus plebeius* [16]. In the definitive host, the parasitic organism creates eggs that hatch into first period larvae (L1), which are expelled with faeces, eaten by slugs and become infective third period larvae (L3). L3 are then expelled through mucoid secretions of the slug and pollute soil and vegetables [16]. Definitive host and man get infected with consuming polluted vegetables or even the infected slugs themselves. L3 migrate through lymphatic system and arrive inside the mesenteric artery, where they become adults [16]. In man, the worm can reach this adult egg-laying period, but larvae are trapped inside granulomas in the intestinal wall and cannot evolve, hence, man is a dead-lock for *A. costaricensis* [16]. Presently, *A. costaricensis* is an illustration of an hemi-zoonosis (the parasitic organism cannot go back from man to animals) of the biological pattern [16].

2. Pathophysiology of Angiostrongyliasis

Angiostrongyliasis is a parasitic disease that is caused by the ingestion of contaminated raw snail or slug, the intermediate host. The term angiostrongylosis, or angiostrongyliasis, if used without the adjective, also might give rise to confusion, since the same term is applied to the pulmonary infection of dogs by A. vasorum and might be used for infection by any other Angiostrongylus species [1]. Even the term cerebral or ocular angiostrongyliasis might prove in the future to pose similar disadvantages [1]. The scientifically correct term angiostrongyliasis cantonensis poses been used recently [1].

In 1982, Yoshimura et al. studied the history of *A. cantonensis* infection in athymic nude and neonatally thymectomized mice [18]. In this work, BALB/c athymic nude and thymus-reconstituted nude mice and neonatally thymectomized BALB/c mice were infected with third period larvae of *A. cantonensis* and the worm burdens of the mice were determined at various times after infection [18]. Yoshimura et al. found that when the nude and thymectomized mice were exposed to the parasitic organism, some worms were found to migrate from the brain to lungs but died there without reaching maturity and this pulmonary arterial migration of the worms in the nude did not occur following thymic reconstitution [18]. Yoshimura et al suggested that the inability of murine intracranial worms to migrate to the lungs was at least in part owing to thymus-dependent mechanisms, and also that the failure of worm maturation in mouse lungs might be owing to thymus-independent immune mechanisms and/or nonimmunological mechanisms [18].

After the recent discovery of *A. costaricensis*, another rat parasitic organism causing human disease in Costa Rica, it becomes needed to distinguish between angiostrongyliasis cantonensis (eosinophilic meningitis) and angiostrongyliasis costaricensis (intra-abdominal eosinophilic granulomatosis) [1]. *A. cantonensis* was named *Pulmonema cantonensis* by its discoverer and later was described under the name *Haemostrongylus ratti* [1].

3. Clinical Presentation

According to the study of Hwang and Chen on special clinical characteristics of *A. cantonensis* among 82 pediatric population in Taiwan, 87% could be traced to a history of contact with the intermediate host, the giant African snail, *A. fulica,* which played a main role in transmission [19]. They noted that the incubation period (average: 13.2 days) was shorter in pediatric population than in adults and in about one-third (30.5%) of the total scenarioes, the clinical form was meningoencephalitis, which was higher than in adult scenarioes seen in Thailand [19]. Hwang and Chen said that the most common clinical symptom was fever (91.5%), followed by vomiting and headache [19]. In addition, the percentages of sixth and seventh cranial neuropathy related with the disease were 19.5% and 11.0% respectively [19]. In this study, ophthalmologic fundoscopy showed that 25.0% with papilledema, which was significantly higher than seen in adults in Thailand [19]. In, 2001, Tsai et al. done a retrospective cohort study among Thai laborers with eosinophilic meningitis who ate raw snails (*A. canaliculatus*), as well as an environmental surveillance of larvae in snails [20]. In this series, central nervous system presentations included headache, fever, Brudzinski's sign/stiff neck, hyperesthesia, cranial nerve palsy, diplopia, and ataxia whereas laboratory findings included peripheral eosinophilia and cerebrospinal fluid eosinophilia; elevated immunoglobulin (Ig) E levels; and transient expands in white blood cell count and in serum levels of creatine kinase, transaminase, and lactate dehydrogenase [20]. Tsai et al. mentioned that the severity of disease and eosinophilia were correlated with the number of ingested snails and meningeal and basal ganglion enhancement was noted on magnetic resonance imaging in several affected cases [20]. The prognosis of neurologic angiostrongyliasis is usually good; however, fatal and chronic scenarioes do occur [4].

Ocular angiostrongyliasis is another clinical presentation. Ocular angiostrongyliasis is sporadically reported in the endemic setting. Usually, ocular angiostrongyliasis occurs concordant with meningitis [21 - 22], however, it occasionally occurs without meningitis [23]. In 1986, Singalavanija et al. reported a case of intravitreal angiostrongyliasis in a Thai female who had eaten raw snails [24]. In this case, after immobilising the worm by use of an intravitreal cryoprobe it was successfully removed via the pars plana with vitreous foreign body forceps [24].

Diagnosis of Angiostrongyliasis

For angiostrongyliasis, direct clinical or laboratory evidence of the etiologic agent is usually not set because reliable tests are not yet available. Eosinophilic pleocytosis is the main laboratory finding [4, 25]. Occasionally, living larvae can be identified histologically in the cerebrospinal fluid (CSF), eye, or other tissue [4]. In 2005, Kumar et al recently reported their successful removal of a live *A. cantonensis* from the anterior chamber [26]. According to the report of Hwang and Chen, most of the scenarioes in this study had peripheral leukocytosis (above $10{,}000/mm^3$) and eosinophilia (above 10%); the percentages were 82.9% and 84.1%, respectively [19]. The worm recovery rate from cerebrospinal fluid by lumbar puncture of 82 scenarioes was 41.5%; 141 worms were collected from one female affected case using a pumping mean [19].

The immunological diagnosis becomes the useful alternative diagnostic technique. Although the diagnosis of neurologic angiostrongyliasis is usually made clinically, serologic means including ELISA (enzyme-connected immunosorbent tool) can be helpful [4]. In 1986, Chen evaluated metabolic and purified antigens of adult or juvenile *A. cantonensis* by ELISA and compared against *Toxocara canis* antigen for sensitivity and specificity [27]. In this study, sera and CSF from both rats and man gave higher ELISA values against antigens of *A. cantonensis* than those obtained from negative control samples [27]. Chen showed that cross reaction occurred between *T. canis* and *A. cantonensis* and noted that of four *A. cantonensis* antigens tested, a Sephacryl S-300 'purified' fraction was shown to be superior in the ELISA to determine angiostrongyliasis [27]. In 1984, Bhopale et al detected serum antibodies in suspected angiostrongyliasis affected case by ELISA [28]. In this study, the antibody titre was 1:51,200 in the serum and 1:6,400 in CSF with preadult *A. cantonensis* antigen [28]. In addition, other tests like AGD and CIEP failed to show any positive reaction with both preadult and adult worm antigens [28]. In 2002, Intapan et al studied specific IgG antibody subclasses to *A. cantonensis* in affected cases with angiostrongyliasis [29]. In this study, total IgG, IgG1, IgG2, IgG3, IgG4, IgA and IgM specific antibodies against *A. cantonensis* somatic antigen were determined by ELISA in sera from proven human angiostrongyliasis scenarioes, clinically suspected angiostrongyliasis scenarioes with eosinophilic meningitis and healthy control [29]. According to this study, main differences were evident in the distributed apperance of the IgG subclass antibodies between the affected case groups [29]. The IgG1 antibody demonstrated the highest sensitivity and specificity whereas the IgM and IgA responses were generally poor in both affected case groups and the levels of the specific IgG antibody subclasses possibly imply immune responses to the parasitic organism [29].

Pathology and Complication

Concerning pathology of angiostrongyliasis, Sonakul described pathology in 4 mortality scenarioes [30]. In this case series, there was infiltration of the meninges and around intracerebral vessels by varying proportions of lymphocytes, plasma cells and eosinophils [30]. Numerous tracks and microcavities were found in the brains, and in the spinal cords, varying in size and in age, with older tracks containing debris and gitter cells, newer tracks showing disruption of brain tissue, with and without haemorrhage [30]. Sonakul noted that numerous fourth and fifth period Angiostrongylus larvae, alive and dead, were found in the meninges and brain tissue, occasionally in blood vessels or perivascular spaces [30]. In addition, cellular reaction was more often related with dead larvae [30]. In 1988, Yoshimura et al. suggested that CSF eosinophils released granule constituents into the outside of the cells and these secretion products could interact with the intracranial worms and were probably related to worm mortality [31]. As degenerative atrophy or partial loss of Purkinje cells and the spongy vacuolation of the white matter were noted in the cerebellum of infected mice, they suggested that CSF eosinophils could be a possible cause of neurological disorders in *A. cantonensis* [31]. Recently, Chen et al noted that that matrix metalloproteinase-9

(MMP-9)/tissue inhibitors of metalloproteinases-1 (TIMP-1) imbalance in angiostrongyliasis might be related with eosinophilic meningitis [32]. They found that Elevated MMP-9 mRNA expression coincided with protein levels and proteolytic activity, as demonstrated by means of positive immunoreactivity and gelatin zymography and CSF protein contents correlated significantly with MMP-9 intensity and CSF eosinophilia [32]. Wang and Wan said that magnetic resonance imaging was helpful in deliningesting the problematic lesions during the acute pposese of angiostrongyliasis caused by *A. cantonensis* [33]. However, they noted that immunologic responses in the central nervous system at the early period of angiostrongyliasis were not sufficient to be observed by image studies [33]. Although the outcome of angiostrongyliasis is usually benign mortality poses been reported as the most serious complication [1 – 2].

Considering abdominal angiostrongyliasis, three fundamental histopathological findings can be detected microscopically: (1) a massive infiltration of eosinophils in all layers of the intestinal wall, (2) a granulomatous reaction and (3) eosinophilic vasculitis affecting arteries, veins, lymphatics and capillaries [34].Graeff-Teixeira et al. concluded that observation of this histopathological triplet excluded other causes of "eosinophilic gastroenteritis" and establishes the diagnosis of probable abdominal angiostrongyliasis [34].

Therapy

There is no specific therapy for this disease [4]. Corticosteroids might be useful to relieve expanded intracranial pressure [4]. The lumbar puncture also provides symptomatic relief [1 – 2]. The role of anthelmintic drugs, such thiabendazole and ivermectin, is not yet known [4]. Recently, Lai et al. studied efficacy of albendazole-GM6001 co-therapy against *A. cantonensis*-induced meningitis in BALB/c mice [35]. In this work, co-administration of drugs created marked effects; to kill the infecting larvae and to block MMP-9 activity and the combination therapy minimized MMP-9 activity by 89.2% in cerebrospinal fluid [35]. Lai et al found that the numbers of inflammatory cells expanded significantly upon establishment of infection, but subsided upon co-therapy and significantly fewer larvae were recovered from treated mice than from untreated, infected mice [35]. Lai et al. strongly suggested that co-therapy with albendazole and GM6001 might be an useful approach for the therapy of human angiostrongyliasis [35]. Recently, Mentz and Graeff-Teixeira said that drug therapy was a challenge since the worms and its evolving larvae live or migrate inside vessels and efficient killing of the parasitic organisms might create more severe problematic lesions [36]. They noted that larvicidal effect of certain drugs appeared to be more easily accomplished but this outcome was not useful in abdominal angiostrongyliasis since clinical presentations appear to result from sexual maturation of the worms [36]. Mentz and Graeff-Teixeira reviewed the drug trials in murine researchal models and concluded that most of them could not be considered good candidates for therapy of human infection, except for PF1022A, pyrantel and flubendazole [36].

Prevention

Prevention of the angiostrongyliasis can be easily done based on the principle of basic food sanitation. The deep-rooted habit as ingestion of raw and poorly uncooked fresh water crab and crayfish should be corrected. Health education is needed. Surveillance of the contamination of the infective period larvae in the fresh water intermediate hosts is also important preventive mean. There are many epidemiological investigations on the contamination of the infective period larvae in the fresh water intermediate hosts in many endemic countries. Owing to the study of Pipitgool et al. a survey of Angiostrongylus infections in rats and snails was carried out in the provinces of Ubon Ratchathani, Udon Thani. Kalasin, Chaiyaphum and Khon Kaen in northeast Thailand [37]. In this work, only two *Rattus norvegicus* and one *Bandicota indica* out of 151 *R. rattus*, 52 *R. norvegicus* and 69 *B. indica* examined were infected with adult lung worms and all worms recovered were *A. cantonensis* [37]. Prevalence of infection in 423 *Pila polita* was 0.9% whereas all of 77 *P. ampullacea* were negative for larvae [37]. This report was also the first proven finding of A. malaysiensis in northeast Thailand [37]. Conclusively, proper preparation of food, control of mollusks and planarians, and elimination of rodents are important measures in limiting the further spread of eosinophilic meningitis caused by *A. cantonensis* [4].

References

[1] Jindrak K. Angiostrongyliasis cantonensis (eosinophilic meningitis, Alicata's disease). *Contemp. Neurol. Ser.* 1975;12:133-64.

[2] Takeuchi T. Angiostrongyliasis. Ryoikibetsu Shokogun Shirizu. 1999;(24 Pt 2):474-6.

[3] Bhaibulaya M. Snail borne parasitic zoonoses: angiostrongyliasis. *Southeast Asian J. Trop. Med. Public. Health.* 1991;22 Suppl:189-93.

[4] Koo J, Pien F, Kliks MM. Angiostrongylus (Parastrongylus) eosinophilic meningitis. *Rev. Infect. Dis.* 1988;10:1155-62.

[5] Scrimgeour EM. Distributed apperance of Angiostrongylus cantonensis in Papua New Guinea. *Trans R. Soc. Trop. Med Hyg.* 1984;78:776-9.

[6] Scrimgeour EM, Welch JS. Angiostrongylus cantonensis in East New Britain, Papua New Guinea. *Trans R Soc. Trop. Med. Hyg.* 1984;78:774-5.

[7] Liat LB, Fong YL, Krishnansamy M, Ramachandran P, Mansor S. Freshwater snail consumption and angiostrongyliasis in Malaya. *Trop. Geogr. Med.* 1978;30:241-6.

[8] Lo Re V 3rd, Gluckman SJ. Eosinophilic meningitis owing to Angiostrongylus cantonensis in a returned traveler: case report and review of the literature. *Clin. Infect. Dis.* 2001;33:e112-5.

[9] Bartschi E, Bordmann G, Blum J, Rothen M. Eosinophilic meningitis owing to Angiostrongylus cantonensis in Switzerland. *Infection.* 2004;32:116-8.

[10] Mahajan RK, Almeida AJ, Sengupta SR, Renapurkar DM. Seasonal intensity of Angiostrongylus cantonensis in the intermediate host, Laevicaulis alte. *Int. J. Parasitol.* 1992;22:669-71.

[11] Yen CM, Chen ER, Cheng CW. A survey of Ampullarium canaliculatus for natural infection of Angiostrongylus cantonensis in south Taiwan. *J. Trop. Med. Hyg.* 1990;93:347-50.

[12] Joshua GW, Chuang RY, Cheng SC, Lin SF, Tuan RS, Wang CC. The spliced leader gene of Angiostrongylus cantonensis. *Mol. Biochem. Parasitol.* 1991;46:209-17.

[13] Wang JJ, Lee JD, Chang JH, Chung LY, Chen ER, Yen CM. The susceptibility of five stains mice to infections with Angiostrongylus cantonensis. Gaoxiong Yi Xue Ke Xue Za Zhi. 1995;11:599-603.

[14] Sawabe K, Makiya K. Genetic variability in isozymes of Angiostrongylus malaysiensis. *Southeast Asian J. Trop. Med. Public Health.* 1994;25:728-36.

[15] Arcari M, Baxendine A, Bennett CE. Angiostrongylus cantonensis. Available at http://www.soton.ac.uk/~ceb/Diagnosis

[16] Mojon M. Huma*n angiostrongyliasis caused by Angiostrongylus costaricensis.* Bull. Acad. Natl .Med. 1994;178:625-31.

[17] Morera P, Cespedes R. Angiostrongylus costaricensis n. sp. (Nematoda: Metastrongyloidea), a new lungworm occuring in man in Costa Rica. 1971. *Rev. Biol. Trop.* 2002;50:783-96.

[18] Yoshimura K, Sato K, Uchida K, Oya H. The history of Angiostrongylus cantonensis infection in athymic nude and neonatally thymectomized mice. Z Parasitic organismnkd. 1982;67:217-26.

[19] Hwang KP, Chen ER. Clinical studies on angiostrongyliasis cantonensis among pediatric population in Taiwan. Southeast Asian J Trop Med Public Health. 1991;22 Suppl:194-9.

[20] Tsai HC, Liu YC, Kunin CM, Lee SS, Chen YS, Lin HH, Tsai TH, Lin WR, Huang CK, Yen MY, Yen CM. Eosinophilic meningitis caused by Angiostrongylus cantonensis: report of 17 scenarioes. *Am. J. Med.* 2001;111:109-14.

[21] Kanchanaranya C, Punyagupta S. Case of ocular angiostrongyliasis related with eosinophilic meningitis. *Am. J. Ophthalmol.* 1971;71:931-4.

[22] Teekposesaenee C, Ritch R, Kanchanaranya C. Ocular parasitic infection in *Thailand.Rev. Infect. Dis.* 1986;8:350-6.

[23] Toma H, Matsumura S, Oshiro C, Hidaka T, Sato Y. Ocular angiostrongyliasis without meningitis symptoms in Okinawa, Japan. *J. Parasitol.* 2002;88:211-3.

[24] Singalavanija A, Wangspa S, Teschareon S. Intravitreal angiostrongyliasis. *Aust N Z J. Ophthalmol.* 1986;14:381-4.

[25] Wiwanitkit V. Cerebrospinal fluid examination and interpretation. *Buddhachinaraj. Med. J.* 1999; 17: 42 – 52.

[26] Kumar V, Kyprianou I, Keenan JM. Ocular Angiostrongyliasis: removal of a live nematode from the anterior chamber. *Eye.* 2005;19:229-30.

[27] Chen SN. Enzyme-connected immunosorbent tool (ELISA) for the detection of antibodies to Angiostrongylus cantonensis. *Trans. R. Soc. Trop Med. Hyg.* 1986;80:398-405.

[28] Bhopale MK, Limighte LS, Pradhan VR, Renapurkar DM, Sharma KD. Studies on suspected clinical and researchal angiostrongyliasis: serological responses. *J. Hyg. Epidemiol. Microbiol. Immunol.* 1984;29:283-8.

[29] Intapan PM, Maleewong W, Polsan Y, Sawanyawisuth K, Chotmongkol V. Specific IgG antibody subclasses to Angiostrongylus cantonensis in affected cases with angiostrongyliasis. *Asian Pac. J. Allergy Immunol.* 2002;20:235-40.

[30] Sonakul D. Pathological findings in four scenarioes of human angiostrongyliasis. Southeast *Asian J. Trop. Med. Public Health.* 1978;9:220-7.

[31] Yoshimura K, Sugaya H, Kawamura K, Kumagai M. Ultrastructural and morphometric analyses of eosinophils from the cerebrospinal fluid of the mouse and guinea-pig infected with Angiostrongylus cantonensis. *Parasitic organism Immunol.* 1988;10:411-23.

[32] Chen KM, Lee HH, Chou HL, Liu JY, Tsai BC, Lai SC. Upregulation of MMP-9/TIMP-1 enzymatic system in eosinophilic meningitis caused by Angiostrongylus cantonensis. *Int. J. Exp. Pathol.* 2005;86:81-9.

[33] Wang LC, Wan YL. Alteration of antibodies against the fifth-period larvae and changes in brain magnetic resonance images in researchally infected rabbits with Angiostrongylus cantonensis. *J. Parasitol.* 2004;90:1193-6.

[34] Graeff-Teixeira C, Camillo-Coura L, Lenzi HL. Histopathological criteria for the diagnosis of abdominal angiostrongyliasis. *Parasitol. Res.* 1991;77:606-11.

[35] Lai SC, Jiang ST, Chen KM, Hsu JD, Shyu LY, Lee HH. Efficacy of albendazole-GM6001 co-therapy against Angiostrongylus cantonensis-induced meningitis in BALB/c mice. *Acta Trop.* 2005;93:267-73.

[36] Mentz MB, Graeff-Teixeira C. Drug trials for therapy of human angiostrongyliasis. *Rev. Inst .Med. Trop. Sao Paulo.* 2003;45:179-84.

[37] Pipitgool V, Sithithaworn P, Pongmuttasaya P, Hinz E. Angiostrongylus infections in rats and snails in northeast Thailand. Southeast *Asian J. Trop. Med. Public Health.* 1997;28 Suppl 1:190-3.

Chapter 7

Round Worm Infestation 2: Capillariasis

Introduction to Capillariasis

The nematode (roundworm) *Capillaria philippinensis* is the causative agent of human intestinal capillariasis [1 - 2]. It was first discovered in the Philippines in 1963.

The life cycle involves freshwater fish as intermediate hosts and fish-ingesting birds as definitive hosts [1 – 3]. Embryonated eggs from feces fed to fish hatch and grow as larvae in the fish intestines [1 – 3]. Infective larvae fed to fish-ingesting birds develop into adults [1 – 3]. Larvae become adults in 10 to 11 days, and the first-generation females create larvae [1 – 3]. These larvae develop into males and egg-producing female worms [1 – 3]. Eggs pass with the feces, reach water, embryonate, and infect fish [1 – 3]. Autoinfection is part of the life cycle and causes hyperinfection. Human beings are infected by ingesting small freshwater fish raw [1 – 2]. The parasitic organism multiplies, and symptoms of diarrhea, borborygmus, abdominal pain, and edema develop [1 – 3]. Chronic infections lead to malnutrition, malabsorption, and hence to protein and electrolyte loss, and mortality results from irreversible effects of the infection [1 – 3].

Therapy presents electrolyte replacement and administration of an antidiarrheal agent and mebendazole or albendazole [3]. Presently, *C. philippinensis* is considered a zoonotic disease of migratory fish-ingesting birds [3]. The eggs are disseminated along flyways and infect the fish, and when fish are eaten raw, the disease develops [3].

Epidemiology of Capillariasis

Capillariasis is an important food-borne parasitic zoonosis that is endemic mainly in Asian countries where some people prefer to eat raw freshwater fish. Intestinal capillariasis caused by *C. philippinensis* appeared first in the Philippines and subsequently in Thailand, Japan, Iran, Egypt, and Taiwan, but most infections occur in the Philippines and Thailand [3]. As set researchally, the life cycle involves freshwater fish as intermediate hosts and fish-ingesting birds as definitive hosts [3]. There are many epidemiological studies on capillariasis in Southeast Asia. In Thailand, the first case report of *C. philippinensis* infection poses been published since 1973 by Pradatsundarasar et al. [4]. Since the first case report, there pose been sporadic case reports of the *C. philippinensis* in Thailand [1 - 2, 5 – 8]. In the Philippines, the capillariasis is still an important food-borne parasitic zoonosis at present [9]. In 2000, Belizario et al. reported a 20 year old female from Compostela Valley Province in the Philippines, presenting with chronic diarrhea, borborygmi, bipedal edema, anorexia, and weight loss was seen at Davao Regional Hospital [10]. Considering, further investigation on the etiology of the disease outbreak in symptomatic affected cases in the setting where this affected case lived, 22.2% of individuals tested positive for *C. philippinensis*; infection [10]. Ocular inspection, interviews and focus group discussions revealed that people are fond of ingesting kinilaw or raw fish and they also eat raw shrimps, crabs and snails [10]. Furthermore, the people defecate in the field or in the same body of water where they get the fishes, shrimps, crabs and snails that they eat, thus completing the life cycle of *C. philippinensis*, hence, fish-ingesting birds were likely to pose spread this parasitic organism to the setting [10]. Belizario et al. mentioned that this was the first report of a capillariasis outbreak in Compostela Valley Province, and this should alert health authorities to consider embarking on serious efforts for developing proficiency of laboratory and clinical diagnosis especially in government health facilities where the poor and marginalized sectors of society were likely to consult [10].

Capillariasis is occasionally reported in non-endemic setting. Bird is believed to play an important role in the wide distributed apperance of disease. Since small freshwater and brackish water fish are considered to be the natural intermediate hosts, and fish-ingesting birds potential definitive hosts, Cross suggested that the spread of the parasitic organism might be attributable to migratory birds [11]. A fish-bird life-cycle is thought to be occurring throughout Asia but intestinal capillariasis is reported only in settings where the human population eats raw freshwater fish [12]. Owing to the concept of travel medicine [13], the capillariasis should be concerned in any travelers back from traveling in Thailand and the Philippines. Dronda et al. reported a case of human intestinal capillariasis in a young Colombian man who presented with abdominal pain and not severe, self-limited diarrhea [14]. In this case, Capillaria eggs were visualized in the feces, and therapy with mebendazole (200 mg/d for 3 weeks) resulted in clinical and parasitological cure. Dronda et al. noted that this was the first case in a South American person and the second case reported in Europe, and this case highlighted the acquisition of endemic intestinal parasitosis far away from classically considered settings of endemicity [14].

Concerning the seasoned effect on the prevalence of Capillaria, there is no report concerning *C. philippinensis* but there is a report considering *C. contorta* [15]. In 1991, Yadav and Tandon mentioned for the the role of the climate in the distributed apperance and in regulating populations of *C. contorta* in fowls in India.

Genetic and Molecular Biology of Capillariasis

The basic knowledge on genetic and molecular biology of capillariasis is very limited. There was a report on the mitochondrial DNA polymorphism within and among species of *C. sensu lato* from Australian marsupials and rodents in 2000 [16]. In this work, the nucleotide variation in a mitochondrial DNA (mtDNA) fragment within and among species of *C. sensu lato* from Australian marsupials and rodents was analyzed using a mutation scanning/sequencing approach and the fragment of the cytochrome c oxidase subunit I (COI) was amplified by PCR from parasitic organism DNA, and analysed by sole-strand conformation polymorphism (SSCP) and sequencing [16]. Zhu et al. indicated that the species of *C. sensu lato* examined, although highly variable in their host and tissue specificity, might exhibit the greatest degree of specificity at the level of host genus [16].

Pathophysiology and Clinical Presentation

1. Basic Knowledge on the Pathogenic organism

Capillaria spp is classified in nematode group. Of several species, *C. philippinensis* is the main problematic parasitic organism to human. Capillariasis cause malabsorption of many important nutrients [17]. Separation of true malabsorption caused by a particular parasitic organism from other factors that might coexist with and even mimic malabsorption, including malnutrition, might be very difficult [17]. It should be noted that *C. philippinensis* is now recognized as an important cause of diarrhea in Asia [18]. In addition to *C. philippinensis*, *C. hepatica* is another new emerging zoonosis [19]. The genuine and spurious infections of *C. hepatica* in human beings as well as its infection in rats around the world are widely discussed [20]. The *C. hepatica* eggs were light yellowish-brown in color, 40-60 microns in length and 25-35 microns in width with a 3-4 microns thick shell and two colorless egg plugs 5-9 x 5-8 microns [20]. . The diagnosis of this parasitosis caused by *C. hepatica* is usually made by needle biopsy of the liver in the affected cases who presented with a triad of persistent fever, hepatomegaly and hypereosinophilia, and the affected cases usually recover completely after therapy with thiabendazole [21].

Concerning the life cycle of *C. philippinensis*, it is a parasitic organism of the human small intestine [22]. The male and female worms measure about 4 mm in length, and the females create eggs and juveniles (larvae) that are passed in the human's feces [22]. The eggs embryonate when they reach water, and they are eaten by fish [22]. The eggs hatch in the fish, and the juveniles mature into infective forms in a few weeks [22]. According to the route of transmission, freshwater and brackish-water fish might act as the intermediate host of the parasitic organism [23]. The definitive host is infected when it eats the fish containing infective juveniles [22]. As in the case with *Strongyloides stercoralis*, the juveniles that are passed by females can reinfect the host directly (autoinfection), so massive infections with this parasitic organism are possible [22]. Heavy infections with this parasitic species cause serious damage to the lining of the small intestine resulting in symptoms including diarrhea, abdominal cramps, malaise, etc [22].

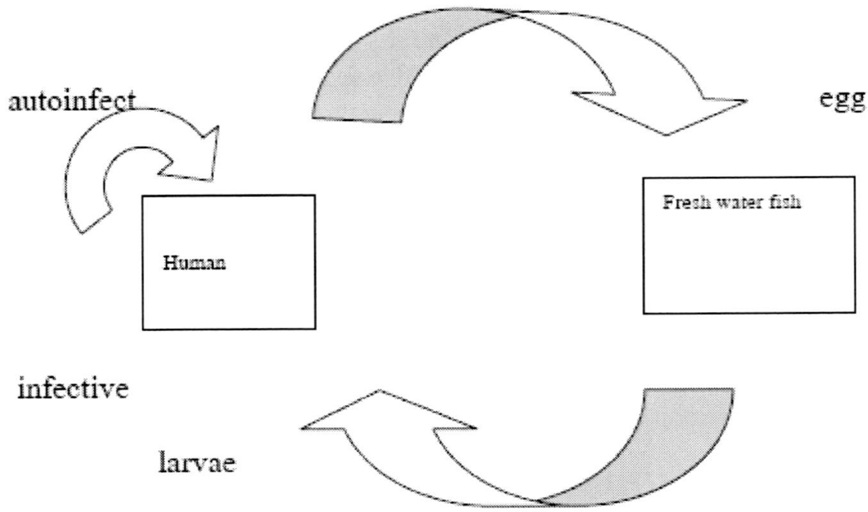

Wiwanitkit V, 2005

Figure 1. Diagram for life cycle of *C. philippinensis*.

2. Pathophysiology of Capillariasis

Capillariasis is a parasitic disease that is caused by the ingestion of contaminated raw fish, the intermediate host. Presently, it is of interest in that the eggs might be confused with the eggs of trichuris [24]. Most scenarioes had intermittent or continuous voluminous watery diarrhea for one month to three years with hypoalbuminemia [25]. Borborygmi, vague abdominal pain, weight loss and pedal edema were significant related symptoms [25].

For *C. hepatica*, Borucinska et al. studied clinicopathological features and histopathology of researchal hepatic capillariasis in muskrats (*Ondatra zibethicus*) [26]. In this work, food intake, body weight, and selected clinicopathological parameters were measured every 2 days for 28 days in the short-term study and every 14 days for 184 days in the long-term study [26]. According to this study, muskrats in the short-term study had moderate to severe necrotizing granulomatous hepatitis related with not severe anorexia and weight loss, varying degrees of leukocytosis with eosinophilia and elevation of serum alanine and aspartate aminotransferases [26]. No significant changes in packed cell volume, hemoglobin, total plasma protein, albumin, blood urea nitrogen, bilirubin, lactate dehydrogenase or alkaline phosphatase were found among animals from the short-term study whereas muskrats in the long-term study had severe necrotizing granulomatous hepatitis related with marked anorexia, weight loss and 60% fatality over 39 days post-inoculation [26]. In addition, hepatic problematic lesions at 184 days post-inoculation consisted of minimal to severe liver replacement by *C. hepatica* eggs [26].

3. Clinical Presentation

According to the study of Bair et al. in Taiwan in 2004, its clinical symptoms are characterized by chronic diarrhea, abdominal pain, borborygmus, marked weight loss, protein and electrolyte loss and cachexia [27]. For intestinal capillariasis, intestinal mucosal abnormalities might be present but the diagnoses are usually made on criteria other than small bowel biopsy [28].

Diagnosis of Capillariasis

For capillariasis, direct clinical or laboratory evidence of the etiologic agent is usually by microscopic mean. The determination of the *C. philippinensis* in the affected cases' stool is the clue for diagnosis of intestinal capillariasis. Morphologically, the unembryonated eggs *C. philippinensis* are peanut shaped and are usually between 25-45μm long and 20 - 25 μm wide. Additional gastroduodenoscopy can show normal jejunal mucosa although histology revealed flattened villi, crypt proliferation, acute inflammation, and eosinophilic granulomata [29].

The immunological diagnosis becomes the useful alternative diagnostic technique. In 1975, Banzon et al. studied the serology of *C. philippinensis* infection on reactivity of human sera to antigens prepared from *C. obsignata* and other helminths [30]. In this work, the reactivity of sera from 151 confirmed human scenarioes of Capillaria philippinensis infection was examined by double diffusion and indirect hemagglutination (IHA) tests chiefly against *C. obsignata* antigen because of the present unavailability of *C. philippinensis* antigen and antigens from additional parasitic organisms and other human and animal sera representing a variety of helminthic infections were used for comparison [30]. Of 71 pre-therapy human sera, 56.3% were reactive by double diffusion test and 85.9% by IHA test with *C. obsignata* antigen and *C. philippinensis* sera were also reactive with *Trichinella spiralis* and *Trichuris vulpis* antigens but not with *Schistosoma japonicum* antigens [30]. According to this study, with *C. obsignata* antigen, IHA titers in human *C. philippinensis* sera are apparently not related to clinical severity of the disease; the titers remain at fairly stable levels during the history of the disease but might tend to decrease after chemotherapy [30]. Banzon et al. noted that the cross-reactivities observed dictated caution in the use and interpretation of any serologic procedure for human intestinal capillariasis; nevertheless, the IHA test using *C. obsignata* antigen might be a useful additional tool in the study of *C. philippinensis* infection both for clinical and epidemiologic purposes especially when the efficiency of stool examination was decreased by changes in the reproductive activity of the helminth [30].

Pathology and Complication

Concerning pathology of intestinal capillariasis, the defect in intestinal mucosa is the hallmark pathology [31- 32]. Flattened villi, crypt proliferation, acute inflammation, and eosinophilic granulomata are the main histopathological findings [29]. Small bowel series and colonoscopic study can reveal not severe dilatation and thickened mucosa of jejunum and ileum, which suggested malabsorption [27].

Intestinal capillariasis can pose the most serious complication as mortality whereas the common complication is malabsorption. Pseudo-obstruction of the intestine was also reported [33].

Concerning the hepatic capillariasis, ultrastructural changes in the liver cells showed dysplastic changes and this might be a sequelae of mechanical injury or direct antigenic insult of the parasitic organism or their toxins on the liver cells [34]. According to the study of el Nassery et al in 1996, it was noticed that most of the granulomata were in the fibrotic period denoting acceleration in the process of healing of the problematic lesions and no freshly deposited ova and hence no active cellular granuloma [34].

Therapy

For intestinal capillariasis, adequate therapy with anthelmintics and general management can result in good outcome. Mebendazole and albendazole are the two sucessful drugs of choice [35 – 36]. In 1987, albendazole was used to treat intestinal capillariasis in hospitalized affected cases seen in Northern Luzon in the Philippines in the trial of Cross and Basaca-Sevilla [35]. In initial studies, four affected cases responded satisfactorily to the drug in dosages of 400 mg/day in divided doses for 20 days and this was the same dosage used for mebendazole, which had been the drug of choice in tringesting the parasitosis [35]. In further studies, 16 affected cases with *C. philippinensis*, were treated with 400 mg/day of the drug for 10 days, and 15 were completely cured and the one therapy failure was found to be passing eggs of the parasitic organism three months later, and was retreated with the standard mebendazole regimen of 400 mg/day for 20 days [35]. According to this report, side effects attributed to albendazole were not reported in any of the affected cases [35]. Cross and Basaca-Sevilla proposed that albendazole, 400 mg/day in two divided doses, was the recommended drug of choice in Northern Luzon in the Philippines [35].

For hepatic capillariasis, both mebendazole and albendazole are also the two sucessful drugs of choice. In 1996, El Gebaly et al. studied effect of mebendazole and ivermectin in researchal hepatic capillariasis [37]. In this study, mebendazole and ivermectin were tried during three different pposeses of *C. hepatica* infection [37]. At an early pposese, when immature forms were present both drugs were sucessful in causing destruction and degeneration of the larvae, thus preventing subsequent growth and maturation and consequently the complete absence of eggs [37]. During the second pposese, which is found to be the most critical period the two drugs used led to degeneration and resorption of most of adult worms [37]. In the third pposese both mebendazole and ivermectin were sucessful in decreasing the mean number of eggs [37]. After therapy the topographic changes were in the form of disorganized cuticle of the worms and absence of surface uniformity [37]. El Gebaly et al. mentioned that the effect of the two drugs indicate that both of them were sucessful in the therapy of hepatic capillariasis [37].

Prevention

Prevention of the capillariasis can be easily done based on the principle of basic food sanitation. The deep-rooted habit as ingestion of raw and poorly uncooked fresh water fish should be corrected. Health education is needed. Surveillance of the contamination of the infective period larvae in the fresh water intermediate hosts is also an important preventive mean. However, the available document on this topic is rather limited.

References

[1] Kunaratanapruk S, Iam-Ong S, Chatsirimongkol C. Intestinal capillariasis. *Ramathibodi Med. J.* 1981; 4 : 206 – 13.

[2] Pathnacharoen S, Tansupposeswadikul S, Manutstitt S, Thanangkul B. Intestinal capillariasis. *Ramathibodi Med. J.* 1983; 6: 277 – 83.

[3] Cross JH. Intestinal capillariasis. *Clin. Microbiol.Rev.* 1992;5:120-9.

[4] Pradatsundarasar A, Pecharanond K, Chintanawongs C, Ungthavorn P. The first case of intestinal capillariasis in Thailand. *Southeast Asian J. Trop. Med. Public Health.* 1973;4:131-4.

[5] Tesana S, Bhuripanyo K, Sanpitak P, Sithithaworn P. Intestinal capillariasis from Udon Thani Province, Northeastern part of Thailand. *J. Med. Assoc. Thai.* 1983; 66: 128 – 31.

[6] Chayakul P, Ovartlarnporn B, Kulwichit P, Piratvisut T, Kunasakdakun A. Intestinal capillariasis. J Infect Dis Antimicrob Agents. 1988; 5: 187 – 90.

[7] Chitchang S, Chitprasong T, JanTong T, Suksala N. Intestinal capillariasis from Lopburi Province. *R Thai Army Med. J.* 1979; 32: 163 – 5.

[8] Muangmanee L, Aswapokee N, Vanasin B. Intestinal capillariasis. Siriraj Hosp Gaz. 1977; 29: 439 – 45.

[9] Eduardo SL. Food-borne parasitic zoonoses in the Philippines. *Southeast Asian J. Trop. Med. Public Health.* 1991 Dec;22 Suppl:16-22.

[10] Belizario VY, de Leon WU, Esparar DG, Galang JM, Fantone J, Verdadero C. Compostela Valley: a new endemic focus for Capillariasis philippinensis. *Southeast Asian J. Trop. Med. Public Health.* 2000;31:478-81.

[11] Cross JH. Intestinal capillariasis. Parasitol Today. 1990;6:26-8.

[12] Cross JH, Basaca-Sevilla V. Researchal transmission of Capillaria philippinensis to birds. *Trans R Soc. Trop. Med. Hyg.* 1983;77:511-4.

[13] Wiwanitkit V. Amazing Thailand Year 1998-1999 Tourist's health concepts. Chula. *Med. J.* 1998; 42: 975-984.

[14] Dronda F, Cposes F, Sanz A, Lopez-Velez R. Human intestinal capillariasis in an setting of nonendemicity: case report and review. *Clin. Infect. Dis.* 1993;17:909-12.

[15] Yadav AK, Tandon V. Helminth parasitism of domestic fowl (Gallus domesticus L.) in a subtropical high-rainfall setting of India. Beitr Trop Landwirtsch Veterinarmed. 1991;29:97-104.

[16] Zhu X, Spratt DM, Beveridge I, Haycock P, Gasser RB. Mitochondrial DNA polymorphism within and among species of Capillaria sensu lato from Australian marsupials and rodents. *Int. J. Parasitol.* 2000;30:933-8.

[17] Brasitus TA. Parasitic organisms ana malabsorption. : Am J Med. 1979;67:1058-65.

[18] Tanowitz HB, Weiss LM, Wittner M. Diagnosis and therapy of common intestinal helminths. II: Common intestinal nematodes. *Gastroenterologist.* 1994 ;2:39-49.

[19] Bhattacharya D, Patel AK, Das SC, Sikdar A. Capillaria hepatica, a parasitic organism of zoonotic importance--a brief overview. *J. Commun. Dis.* 1999;31:267-9.

[20] Fan PC, Chung WC, Chen ER. Capillaria hepatica: a spurious case with a brief review. *Kaohsiung J. Med. Sci*. 2000;16:360-7.

[21] Berger T, Degremont A, Gebbers JO, Tonz O. Hepatic capillariasis in a 1-year-old child. *Eur. J .Pediatr.* 1990;149:333-6.

[22] Capillaria Philippinensis. Available at http://www.biosci.ohio-state.edu/~parasitic organism/ capillaria.html

[23] Hwang KP. Human intestinal capillariasis (Capillaria philippinensis) in Taiwan. Zhonghua Min Guo Xiao Er Ke Yi Xue Hui Za Zhi. 1998;39:82-5.

[24] Walden J. Parasitic diseases. Other roundworms. Trichuris, hookworm, and Strongyloides. *Prim. Care.* 1991;18:53-74.

[25] Chunlertrith K, Mairiang P, Sukeepaisarnjaroen W. Intestinal capillariasis: a cause of chronic diarrhea and hypoalbuminemia. *Southeast Asian J. Trop. Med. Public Health.* 1992;23:433-6.

[26] Borucinska JD, Van Kruiningen HJ, Caira JN, Garmendia AE. Clinicopathological features and histopathology of researchal hepatic capillariasis in muskrats (Ondatra zibethicus*). J .Wildl. Dis.* 1997;33:122-30.

[27] Bair MJ, Hwang KP, Wang TE, Liou TC, Lin SC, Kao CR, Wang TY, Pang KK. Clinical features of human intestinal capillariasis in Taiwan. *World J. Gastroenterol.* 2004;10:2391-3.

[28] Brandborg LL. Histologic diagnosis of diseases of malabsorption. *Am. J .Med.* 1979 ;67:999-1006.

[29] Wongsawasdi L, Ukarapol N, Lertprasertsuk N. The endoscopic diagnosis of intestinal capillariasis in a child: a case report. *Southeast Asian J. Trop. Med. Public Health.* 2002;33:730-2.

[30] Banzon TC, Lewert RM, Yogore MG. Serology of Capillaria philippinensis infection: reactivity of human sera to antigens prepared from Capillaria obsignata and other helminths. *Am. J. Trop. Med. Hyg.* 1975;24:256-63.

[31] Sun SC, Cross JH, Berg HS, Kau SL, Singson C, Banzon T, Watten RH. Ultrastructural studies of intestinal capillariasis Capillaria philippinensis in human and gerbil hosts. *Southeast Asian J. Trop .Med. Public Health.* 1974;5:524-33.

[32] Fresh JW, Cross JH, Reyes V, Whalen GE, Uylangco CV, Dizon JJ. Necropsy findings in intestinal capillariasis. *Am. J. Trop. Med. Hyg.* 1972;21:169-73.

[33] Wilairatana P. Capillariasis with chronic intestinal pseudo-obstruction. *Southeast Asian J. Trop. Med. Public Health.* 1994;25:600-2.

[34] el Nassery SF, el Gebaly MW, el Azzouni MZ, Hammouda NA, el Shenawie S, Allam SR. Effect of mebendazole and ivermectin in researchal hepatic capillariasis B: histopathological and ultrastructural studies. *J. Egypt Soc. Parasitol.* 1996;26:315-26.
[35] Cross JH, Basaca-Sevilla V. Albendazole in the therapy of intestinal capillariasis. *Southeast Asian J. Trop .Med. Public Health.* 1987;18:507-10.
[36] Singson CN, Banzon TC, Cross JH. Mebendazole in the therapy of intestinal capillariasis. *Am. J. Trop .Med. Hyg.* 1975;24:932-4.
[37] El Gebaly MW, Nassery SF, El Azzouni MZ, Hammouda NA, Allam SR. Effect of mebendazole and ivermectin in researchal hepatic capillariasis: parasitological, scanning electron microscopy and immunological studies. *J. Egypt Soc. Parasitol.* 1996;26:261-72.

Chapter 8

Round Worm Infestation 3: Gnathostomiasis

Introduction to Gnathostomiasis

Gnathostomiasis is a helminthic zoonotic disease that poses been increasingly reported in travelers returning from the endemic settings. *Gnathostoma spinigerum* is the main causative agent of human gnathostomiasis, a parasitic zoonosis with a great variety of clinical presentations [1 – 3]. Generally, human beings are infected by consumption of third-period larvae (L3) of *G. spinigerum* in infected hosts in the form of partially cooked or uncooked food. In general, this infection is found mainly in Asia and Latin America where raw and pickled fish are part of the diet [4].

It is owing to the consumption of raw or insufficiently cooked meat (chicken, snakes), frogs or fish, contaminated with larvae of the gender Gnathostoma [5]. Once confined primarily to Southeast Asia, gnathostomiasis now is a public health concern in Mexico and other countries [6].

For gnathostomiasis, human is an incidental host. Gnathostomiasis includes a great variety of clinical presentations caused by cutaneous and/or visceral larva migrans syndrome [5]. Some visceral involvement, more specifically neurological forms, might lead to significant morbidity and fatality [7]. The diagnosis is occasionally confirmed by the detection of the Gnathostoma larva in the skin or viscera [7]. Often the diagnosis relies on epidemiological, clinical and biological (hypereosinophilia, positive serologic test) grounds [7].

Epidemiology of Gnathostomiasis

Gnathostomiasis is an important food-borne parasitic zoonosis that is endemic mainly in Asian countries where some people prefer to eat raw freshwater fish [8]. The genus Gnathostoma contains at least twelve distinctive species [9]. Among these, 6 species, namely *G. spinigerum*, *G. hispidum*, *G. doloresi*, *G. vietnamicum*, *G. malaysiae* and *G. nipponicum*, are found in wild animals in Asia [9]. Related to human gnathostomiasis, *G. spinigerum* poses long been believed as the only causative species [9]. Until the early 1980s, all gnathostomiasis scenarioes found in main endemic settings in Asia, including Thailand, China and Japan, were caused by infection with *G. spinigerum* [9]. In the early 1980s in Japan, new gnathostomiasis scenarioes appeared in urban settings and these scenarioes were shown to be caused by *G. hispidum*, of which larvae were found in roaches imported from Taiwan, Korea, or China [9].

Recently, infections with *G. nipponicum* caused by ingesting locally obtained raw fish, were reported in Mie Prefecture, and about ten scenarioes of infection with *G. doloresi*, caused by ingesting raw slices of freshwater fishes, were found in Miyazaki Prefecture [9]. It should be noted that *G. doloresi* pose been found only in Japan, concentrated in Miyazaki Prefecture [10]. So far four Gnathostoma species are responsible for zoonotic infections in human beings [9]. Although most of these affected cases were of cutaneous gnathostomiasis, some affected cases presented to the hospital with unusual clinical presentations including pulmonary gnathostomiasis diagnosed by immunoserological means, and ileus caused by migration of the late 3rd period larva in the colonic tissue, which was found by post-operative histopathological examination [10]. Since *G. hispidum* and *G. doloresi*, like *G. spinigerum*, are widely distributed in Asia, care should be taken with the detection of species causing gnathostomiasis [9]. In 2000, the first human case report of gnathostomiasis owing to *G. malaysiae* was documented by Nomura et al [11]. Until present, five species causing human gnathostomiasis, *G. hispidum*, *G. doloresi*, *G. nipponicum*, *G. spinigerum* and *G. malaysiae* can be distinguished. However, as previously mentioned, most of human gnathostomiasis is caused by *G. spinigerum*.

Gnathostomiasis is rarely reported in travelers, although the disease remains a main public health problem in Southeast Asia. In America, the first recorded case of gnathostomiasis was in Mexico in 1970, and the numbers of gnathostomiasis affected cases in Mexico seems to be increasing dramatically with time [8]. A creeping eruption and Quincke's edema (slowly migrating erythema with pruritus) appeared in travelers who had eaten raw freshwater fish or shrimp and are the clues for further diagnosis [11].

Gnathostomiasis is an helminthic disease of animals owing to a nematode belonging to the gender Gnathostoma. This gender includes many species, the most common being *G. spinigerum*.

Concerning the effect of environment on the gnathostomiasis, in 1989, Rojekittikhun et al.[12] said that the highest intensity of *Gnathostoma* spp L3 in the swamp eels could be detected during the rainy season. Saksirisampant et al. [13]recently mentioned the possible effect of rainfall on the prevalence of eel infection. A recent study on the relation between rainfall (derived from the geographical data) and the prevalence of Gnathostomo spp by Wiwanitkit [14] revealed the least-square equation plot rainfall (y) versus prevalence (x) as $y = 9.68x + 1{,}035.12$ ($r = 0.83$; $p < 0.01$). A significant correlation was discerned between rainfall and the prevalence of eel infection but not for the season of the survey [14]. This study [14] can confirm the effect of rainfall on the prevalence of *Gnathostoma* spp L3 in the swamp eels, which was reported by Saksirisampant *et al* [13]. According to the study by Wiwanitkit, infection prevalence correlated significantly with rainfall but not with season, which could suggest that the prevalence of infections among eels do not depend on season

[14]. Indeed, there was also another report on the effect of season on the intensity but not for the prevalence of eel infection [12]. Similar to the previous study [13], Wiwanitkit concluded that the prevalence of eel infection might depend on rainfall rather than season [14].

Table 1. Epidemiology of human *Gnathostoma* spp

Species	Countries
G. hispidum	Thailand, Viet Nam, Malaysia, Philippines, Korea, Taiwan, China
G. spinigerum	India, Bangladesh, Burma, Thailand, Laos, Cambodia, Viet Nam, Malaysia, Indonesia, Philippines, China, Japan
G. nipponicum	Japan
G. doloresi	India, Burma, Thailand, Viet Nam, Singapore, Philippines, Taiwan, Japan, New Guinea
G. malaysiae	Malaysia

Wiwanitkit V, 2005

Genetic and Molecular Biology of Gnathostomiasis

The basic knowledge on genetic and molecular biology of gnathostomiasis is rather limited. In 2000, Almeyda-Artigas et al. done an interesting study [15]. In this study, from several gnathostome species the complete internal transcribed spacer ITS-2 ribosomal DNA (rDNA) repeat sequence and a fragment of the 5.8S rDNA were obtained by direct polymerase chain reaction cycle-sequencing and silver-staining means [15]. They found that the ITS-2 enabled the differentiation of *G. spinigerum* from Thailand and *G. binucleatum* from Mexico and Ecuador and confirmed the validity of the latter [15]. In addition, they found that the 5.8S rDNA sequences of the 6 Gnathostoma species studied were identical and the results of the ITS-1 agreed with those results of ITS-2 [15]. Leon-Regagnon et al. done another study to clarify the specific identity of the etiological agent of human gnathostomosis in Nayarit State, Mexico by morphological and molecular studies on advanced third period larvae obtained from human and fish tissue [16]. They found that morphological variability did not permit specific detection of the larvae, however, the ITS-2 enabled [16].

Pathophysiology and Clinical Presentation

1 Basic Knowledge on the Pathogenic organism, Gnathostome

Gnathostoma is a genus of parasitic nematodes that occurs in mammals and including human beings. Five species causing human gnathostomiasis, *G. hispidum*, *G. doloresi*, *G. nipponicum*, *G. spinigerum* and *G. malaysiae*, can be distinguished based on the number of nuclei in intestinal epithelial cells of infected larvae, in cross-section [11]. In addition,

Gnathostome larvae can be identified on the basis of other several characteristics: the shape of body, the number of rows of hooklets at the head bulb, the number of hooklets in each row, and the characters with the extension of spines covering the body [17 – 19]. Adult Gnathostoma are usually about 2 to 3 centimeters long and are rust-colored [17]. With respect to morphological structure, third-period larval worms pose been studied more intensively than adults, as it is these larval worms that cause gnathostomiasis. Morphology of the most common species, *G. spinigerum* is well described [1 – 2]. Briefly, the larvae usually pose four rows of hooklets extruding from the surface of the cephalic bulb, which help in lodging into the tissues of their hosts [18]. Tiny cuticular spines run along the length of their bodies. Two types of papillae extend from the worm--a cervical papilla off the main body and two labial papillae on the cephalic bulb [18]. Four sac-like openings in the cephalic bulb generate worm movement by expanding and contracting, and subsequently displacing nearby fluids [18]. L3 worms pose been found ranging in size from approximately 2 millimeters to more than 16 millimeters [18]. The worms pose both a mouth and an anus [18]. At the tip of the cephalic bulb are two lips, through which nutrients are ingested [18].

Concerning the life cycle of *G. spinigerum*, the adult worms live in the stomach or esophagus of the final hosts, dogs and cats [19]. The eggs pass out with the feces, cleave and embryonate in the water in proper temperature [19]. The second period larvae, after molt in embrynoated eggs, are hatched and swim actively in the water, and are ingested by fresh water copepods, including *Mesocyslops leuckarti*, *Eucyclops serrulatus*, *Cyclops strenuus* and *C. vicinus* [19]. The larvae take off the sheath in the digestive tract of the copepod and migrate to the body cavity, to become an early L3 after the second molt [19]. When the copepods are eaten by tadpoles or fishes (the second intermediate host), the early third-period larvae in the digestive tract of the second intermediate hosts enter the muscle, and grow into the advanced third-period larvae [19]. For other species, the life cycles are similar, however, the main difference is the final hosts.

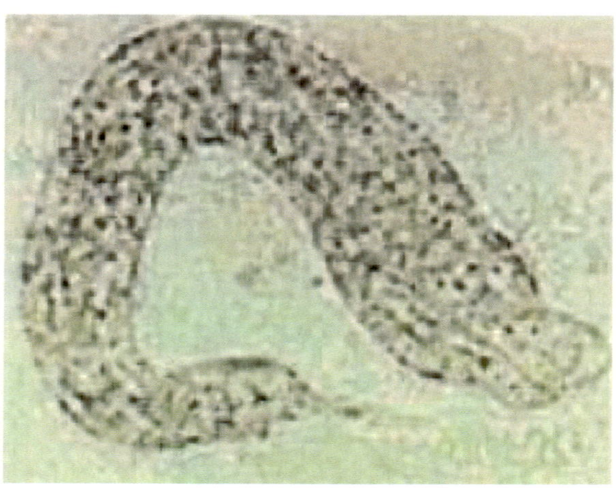

Wiwanitkit V, 2005

Figure 1. Microscopic view of *G. spinigerum*.

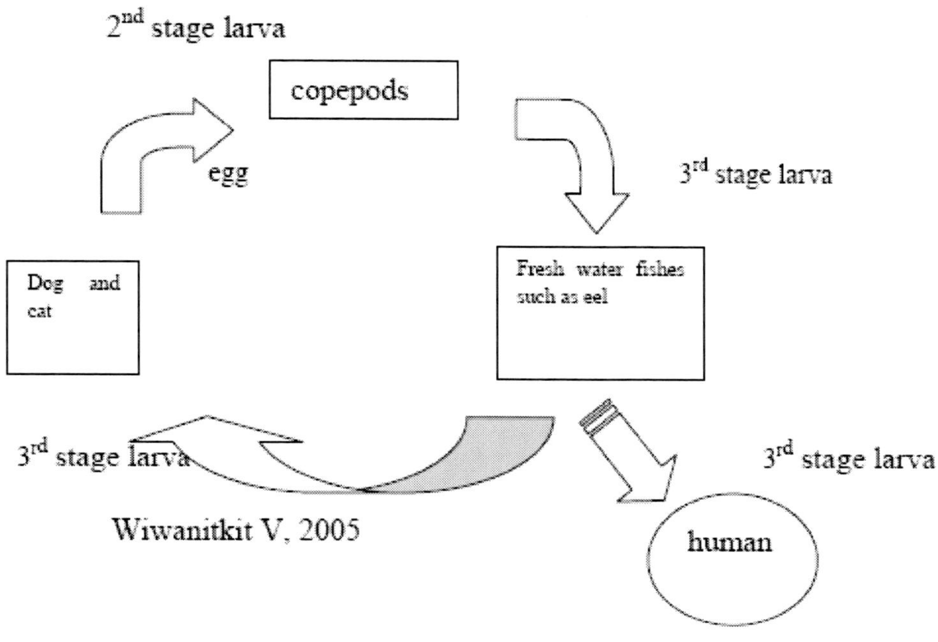

Figure 2. Diagram for life cycle of *G. spinigerum*.

Pigs and wild pigs are documented as final hosts for both *G. hispidum* and *G. doloresi* [19], weasels for *G. nipponicum* [19] and shrimps for *G. malaysiae* [11]. Human beings are infested accidentally by ingestion of contaminated L3 in the second intermediate host, the fresh water fishes.

2. Pathophysiology of Gnathostomiasis

Gnathostomiasis is a systemic parasitic disease that is caused by the ingestion of contaminated raw fish, the intermediate host. Involvement of the skin is a common event, and when it does happen, it can create a superficial or creeping eruption, pseudofurunculosis, and nodular migratory panniculitis [20]. However, the pathophysiology of the human gnathostomiasis is not well described. Magana et al. done a retrospective study of gnathostomiasis and found that the most common skin finding was nodular migratory panniculitis affecting the trunk [20]. In this series, most of the affected cases were males between 20 and 40 years of age [20]. Magana et al. reported that the histopathologic changes were quite characteristic and included: dermal and hypodermal edema with dense mixed infiltrates composed of eosinophils admixed with lymphocytes and neutrophils, eosinophilic vasculitis, flame figures, settings of necrosis, and hemorrhage [20]. Magana et al. said that the existence of these histopathologic features in the context of a clinical picture suggestive of gnathostomiasis permits the pathologist to make the correct diagnosis [20]. For diagnosis, skin tests and antigen-antibody reactions are usually positive for Gnathostoma infection.

The involvement of the neurological system of gnathostomiasis can also be seen. Boongird et al. reviewed the neurological features of the affected cases with nervous system gnathostomiasis and found that the commonest presenting features were radiculomyelitis or radiculomyelitis terminating with encephalitis, and subarachnoid haemorrhage [21]. In this study, the salient feature of the disease was a sudden onset of extremely severe radicular pain and/or headache followed by paralysis of the extremities and/or the cranial nerves and migration signs were also the hallmark of nervous system gnathostomiasis [21]. Boongird et al noted that no sole setting of the nervous system was inaccessible to the highly invasive gnathostome lava and multiplicity and/or rapid progress of problematic lesions beyond the degree of cerebral edema could only be implyed by further migration of the parasitic organism [21]. Boongird et al said that mortality usually occurred from direct extensive involvement of vital centres in the brain stem or from complications including pneumonia or septicaemia [21]. They proposed that multiple cranial nerve palsies were usually bad prognostic signs [21].

For diagnosis, eosinophilia, eosinophilic pleocytosis in the CSF, and a high serum IgE level are noted. Sawanyawisuth et al. said that magnetic resonance (MR) imaging represents a complementary tool for assessing severity and extent of disease [22]. For severe affected scenarioes, MR imaging of the cervical cords showed cord enlargement and diffuse high signal intensity, mainly of the gray-white matter regions [22]. MR imaging of the brain showed hemorrhagic tract and scattered deep intracerebral hemorrhage with diffuse, fuzzy white matter problematic lesions with nodular enhancement [22].

3. Clinical Presentation

Infection status can not be correctly estimated because the gnathostomes are tissue invading nematodes, hence, their infections are not easily diagnosed [19]. Hence, the actual infection rate is hard to calculate [19]. Gnathostomiasis includes a great variety of clinical presentations caused by cutaneous and/or visceral larva migrans syndrome. As previously mentioned, the cutaneous gnathostomiasis is the most common presentation of human gnathostomiasis. The clinical presentation is most commonly characterized by localized, intermittent, migratory swellings of the skin and subcutaneous tissues, often in association with localized pain, pruritus, and erythema [17]. According to the study of Diaz Camacho et al., cutaneous problematic lesions were observed mainly on the face, neck, arms, and legs [23]. They noted that about 70% of the affected cases showed eosinophilia [23]. Characteristically, affected cases with gnathostomiasis pose a moderate to severe elevation of the peripheral eosinophil count, with values not rarely exceeding 50% of the total white blood cell count [17]. Extraction of the worm from the skin following by morphological detection of the gnathostomiasis is also another common diagnostic mean.

Since this worm can migrate to deeper tissues, any organ system might become involved [17]. The central nervous system involvement is common as already mentioned. This tissue nematode involved, because of its high motility, might cause widespread damage in the spinal cord and brain [17]. Clinically, the symptom as migrating radiculopathy, presenting with severe nerve root pain, is a hallmark of gnathostomiasis in the tropical endemic countries including Thailand [24]. The other common symptoms include paralysis of limbs and urinary retention. Less commonly seen are cranial nerve palsies and symptoms of subarachnoid hemorrhage [24]. Eosinophilic meningoradiculomyelitis is also documented [24]. Schmutzhard et al said that the main laboratory finding as eosinophilic pleocytosis in the cerebrospinal fluid, greater than 10%, which in affected cases originating or returning from South-East-Asia, specifically Thailand, was highly suggestive of these parasitic infections [25].

Another important presentation of human gnathostomiasis is ocular gnathostomiasis. Live intraocular nematode is a rare occurrence that is mostly reported in Southeast Asian countries [26 - 27]. The live organism can be successfully removed by vitreous aspiration [27]. Iris holes, uveitis, and subretinal haemorrhage with subretinal tract can be characteristic features of intraocular gnathostomiasis [26]. Detection of this parasitic organism can be made by typical features, which can be identified on light and scanning electron microscopic study [26].

Diagnosis of Gnathostomiasis

Diagnosis of gnathostomiasis is problematic in laboratory medicine. The nature of parasitic organism as tissue invader and its detection is occasionally difficult.

Occasionally, the affected cases can remove larval worms from the skin problematic lesion by pinching with their nails [27]. Subsequently, the parasitic organisms can usually be identified based on morphologic characteristics including number of hooklets on its head-bulb. Albendazole should be administered before incision of the skin problematic lesion when gnathostomiasis was suspected [27].

Concerning the complete blood count, the eosinophilia is common although this finding is not the clue for final diagnosis of human gnathostomiasis. In scenarioes with central nervous system involvement, eosinophilic pleocytosis in the CSF can be seen [24]. The MRI examination can help the diagnosis as previously described. In addition, angiography can also demonstrate mycotic aneurysm typical for cerebral gnathostomiasis [29].

The immunological diagnosis becomes the useful alternative diagnostic technique. Skin test is a common immunological diagnosis for gnathostomiasis. However, a trained medical doctor is required for performing the test and the test provided rather low diagnostic property. hence, other immunological diagnostic technique is developed. ELISA is the acceptable test for diagnostic of gnathostomiasis at present. Suntharasamai et al.. first created an ELISA for immunodiagnosis of human gnathostomiasis using a crude water extract of third-period larvae of *G. spinigerum* as antigen [30]. However, the diagnostic property is not good. ELISA for IgG antibody against the *G. spinigerum* L3 specific protein is recommended. Soogarun et al. [31] noted that fraction III, 24 kd is the specific protein for ELISA development. Soogarun et al. [31] noted that using ultrafiltration technique can help purification of the L3 protein for ELISA development. Nuchprayoon et al [32] noted that the ELISA that detected anti-*G. spinigerum* L3 IgG1 antibody could be a reliable laboratory screening test, whereas anti-*G. spinigerum* L3 IgG2 antibody could be used to confirm the diagnosis. However, the problem of the cross reaction still exists.

Recently Saksirisampant et al. noted that the antibody responses to secreted products (ES) are more closely related to active infection than the anti-whole worm antibody that might persist following the mortality of the parasitic organisms [33]. They also test the using of IgE instead of IgG determination [33]. The overall sensitivity of the ELISA for the IgE antibodies detection were 71.87 per cent and 87.50 per cent with somatic and ES antigens, respectively [33]. For gnathostomiasis of central nervous system, Morakote et al. suggested that parasitic organism-specific antigen might be present on intestinal cell microvilli and cerebrospinal fluid would be a good source of antibodies in studying specificity of antibodies to gnathostome infections [34]. Tuntipopipat et al. suggested that the detection of IgG antibodies in cerebrospinal fluid was more reliable than the the quantitation of IgG antibodies in the paired serum in confirming the diagnosis of cerebral gnathostomiasis [35].

Pathology and Complication

Concerning pathology of cutaneous gnathostomiasis, histopathologic features usually reveal a eosinophilic panniculitis owing to probable larva migrans [36 - 37].

The name "nodular migratory eosinphilic panniculitis" is proposed because of the histopathologic and clinical changes found in infected scenarioes in which the parasitic organisms were found on biopsy [38]. Ollague Torres et al. said that the histological picture was different and changed according to the day the biopsy was taken [39]. For central nervous system infestation, migration signs are also the hallmark of nervous system gnathostomiasis [21]. No sole setting of the nervous system is inaccessible to the highly invasive gnathostome lava [21]. Multiplicity and/or rapid progress of problematic lesions beyond the degree of cerebral edema can only be implyed by further migration of the parasitic organism [21]. Subarachnoid hemorrhage is another common presentation of the nervous gnathostomiasis [40]. However, the finding of the parasitic organism in the cerebrospinal fluid is very rare. For intraocular gnathostomiasis, palpebral edema with conjunctival erythema can develop when problematic lesions developed near the eye [41]. In those scenarioes, routine eye examination usually shows a mobile worm in the anterior chamber [41].

Severe complications of human gnathostomiasis can be seen in the scenarioes with nervous system involvement. Mortality is the most serious outcome and usually related with the subarachnoid hemorrhage [17, 40]. For cutaneous gnathostomiasis, no serious complication is mentioned, with no report on the cutaneous gnathostomiasis as the premalignancy problematic lesion. For ocular gnathostomiasis, the blindness poses never been documented in the literature.

Therapy

For cutaneous gnathostomiasis, albendazole is the classical drugs. In 1992, Kraivichian et al. done interesting clinical trials and found that cure, with no further swelling was seen in 93.9% and 94.1% of the therapy groups, but in none of the placebo group [42]. Additionally, reductions in eosinophil counts and in IG G antibody were observed after therapy [42]. In this study, side effects of albendazole were minimal [42]. Kraivichian et al .concluded that albendazole might be an sucessful compound for the therapy of gnathostomiasis [42]. Suntharasamai et al. noted that during a double-blind randomized placebo control trial evaluating the efficacy of albendazole in cutaneous gnathostomiasis at a dosage of 400 mg twice daily for two weeks, it was observed that gnathostome larvae tended to migrate outward as a result of the therapy so that they could be recovered by excisional biopsy or by picking with a needle [43]. They noted that albendazole could stimulate outward migration of *G. spinigerum* to the dermis in man [43].

Recently, ivermectin is the new drug proposed for therapy of cutaneous gnathostomiasis. Kraivichian et al. found that a sole dose of ivermectin (200 microg/kg) was less sucessful than albendazole (400 mg/day for 21 days) for therapy of cutaneous gnathostomiasis, but there was no statistically significant difference [44].

Nontasut et al done a similar study [45]. They found that comparative therapy of ivermectin and albendazole in affected cases of gnathostomiasis gave the cure at 95.2% and 93.8% respectively [45]. They noted that the ELISA OD and eosinophil counts were minimized after therapy [45]. Nontasut et al. found that side effects in ivermectin were hypotention, dizziness, weakness, and diuresis; side effects of albendazole were nausea, dizziness and expanded alkaline phosphatase [45]. They concluded that ivermectin should be an sucessful drug against gnathostomiasis and more convenient in therapy sole dose [45].

Both albendzaole and ivermectin are also recommended as drugs for therapy of nervous and ocular gnathostomiasis. Recently, Bhende et al. described the use of ultrasound biomicroscopy (UBM) in the detection of an intraocular nematode in a case of suspected nematode-induced uveitis [46]. In this work, UBM was done under topical anesthesia in a affected case with acute painful uveitis suspected to result from an intraocular nematode [46]. Over a 6-minute time span, serial UBM examinations revealed the nematode to move from the iris root into the posterior chamber through the zonules [46]. They concluded that UBM was a useful alternative tool in diagnosis and management of parasitic uveitis [46].

Prevention

Prevention of the gnathostomiasis can be easily done based on the principle of basic food sanitation. The deep-rooted habit of the ingestion of raw and poorly uncooked fresh water fishes should be corrected. Health education is needed. Surveillance of the contamination of the L3 in the fresh water intermediate hosts is also an important preventive mean. There are many epidemiological investigations on the contamination of the L3 in the fresh water intermediate hosts in many endemic countries. Owing to the recent study of Soogarun and Wiwanitkit in Bangkok, the prevalence of *G. spinigerum* L3s in the eels was much higher in the rainy season (June and July, 74%) than during April and Might (8%) [47]. Hence, prevention plans for gnathostomiasis should be empposesized during the rainy season [47]. In a similar study by Saksirisampant et al. prevalence of the infection varied with season, from a high of 38.3% in September to a low of 7.0% in April, being generally high during the rainy season and winter (June-February) [48]. Saksirisampant et al. noted that although the results of an earlier study had indicated that the prevalence of eel infection decreased in November, after the rainy season, the most abrupt decrease observed in the present study occurred at the beginning of summer (March) [48]. However, they proposed that the period covered by their study was unusually wet, and the prevalence of eel infection might depend on rainfall more than season [48]. Similar investigation by Wiwanitkit also revealed that the prevention plans were needed for the period with heavy rainfall [14].

References

[1] Daengsvang S. A monograph on the genus Gnathostoma and gnathostomiasis in Thailand. Tokyo: Southeast Asian Medical Information Center SEAMIC, International Medical Foundation of Japan, 1980:85

[2] Daengsvang S. *Gnathostoma spinigerum* and human gnathostomiasis. A review. In: Sucharit S, eds. The 25th Anniversary of the Faculty of Tropical Medicine, Mahidol University. Bangkok: Krung Siam Press, 1986:124-147

[3] Radomyos P, Daengsvang S. A brief report on *Gnathostoma spinigerum* specimens obtained from human scenarioes. *Southeast Asian J. Trop. Med. Public Health* 1987; 18:215-217

[4] CDC. 1999b. "Gnathostomiasis." Available on: *http://www.dpd.cdc.gov /DPDx /HTML/gnathostomiasis.htm*. Division of Parasitic Diseases, National Center for Infectious Diseases, Centers for Disease Control and Prevention Atlanta, Georgia, 1999

[5] Parola P, Caumes E. Gnathostomiasis. *Med. Trop* .(Mars). 2005;65:9-12.

[6] Ligon BL. Gnathostomiasis: a review of a previously localized zoonosis now crossing numerous geographical boundaries. *Semin. Pediatr. Infect. Dis.* 2005 ;16:137-43.

[7] Clement-Rigolet MC, Danis M, Caumes E. Gnathostomosis, an exotic disease increasingly imported into Western countries. *Presse Med.* 2004;33:1527-32.

[8] Ogata K, Nawa Y, Akahane H, Diaz Camacho SP, Lamothe-Argumedo R, Cruz-Reyes A. Short report: gnathostomiasis in Mexico. *Am J Trop Med Hyg*. 1998 ;58:316-8.

[9] Nawa Y. Historical review and current status of gnathostomiasis in Asia. *Southeast Asian J. Trop. Med. Public Health.* 1991;22 Suppl:217-9.

[10] Nawa Y, Maruyama H, Ogata K. Current status of gnathostomiasis dorolesi in Miyazaki Prefecture, Japan. *Southeast Asian J Trop Med Public Health.* 1997;28 Suppl 1:11-3.

[11] Nomura Y, Nagakura K, Kagei N, Tsutsumi Y, Araki K, Sugawara M. Gnathostomiasis possibly caused by Gnathostoma malaysiae. *Tokai J. Exp. Clin. Med.* 2000;25:1-6.

[12] Rojekittikhun W, Pubampen S, Hiranyachattada P, *et al.* A survey on the infective larvae of *Gnathostoma spinigerum* in fresh water fish sold in the local markets of Bangkok. *J. Trop. Med. Parasitol.* 1989; 12:7-12

[13] Saksirisampant W, Kulkaew K, Nuchprayoon S, Yentakham S, Wiwanitkit V. A survey of the infective larvae of *Gnathostoma spinigerum* in swamp eels bought in a local market in Bangkok, Thailand. *Ann. Trop. Med. Parasitol.* 2002;96:191-5

[14] Wiwanitkit V. A note on the correlation between rainfall and the prevalence of Gnathostoma spp. infective period larvae in swamp eels in Thailand. *Parasitic organism.* 2004 ;11:401-4.

[15] Almeyda-Artigas RJ, Bargues MD, Mas-Coma S. ITS-2 rDNA sequencing of Gnathostoma species (Nematoda) and elucidation of the species causing human gnathostomiasis in the Americas. *J. Parasitol.* 2000;86:537-44.
[16] Leon-Regagnon V, Osorio-Sarabia D, Garcia-Prieto L, Akahane H, Lamothe-Argumedo R, Koga M, Messina-Robles M, Alvarez-Guerrero C. Study of the ethiological agent of gnathostomosis in Nayarit, Mexico. *Parasitol. Int.* 2002 ;51:201-4.
[17] Rusnak JM, Lucey DR. Clinical gnathostomiasis: case report and review of the English-language literature. *Clin. Infect. Dis.* 1993;16:33-5
[18] Morphology of gnathostoma (spinigerum) Available at *http://www.stanford. edu/class /humbio103/Parasitic organisms2001/gnathostomiasis*
[19] Gnathostome. Available at *http://atlas.or.kr/atlas*
[20] Magana M, Messina M, Bustamante F, Cazarin J. Gnathostomiasis: clinicopathologic study. *Am. J. Dermatopathol.* 2004;26:91-5.
[21] Boongird P, Phuapradit P, Siridej N, Chirachariyavej T, Chuahirun S, Vejjajiva A. Neurological presentations of gnathostomiasis. *J. Neurol. Sci.* 1977;31:279-91.
[22] Sawanyawisuth K, Tiamkao S, Kanpittaya J, Dekumyoy P, Jitpimolmard S.
[23] MR imaging findings in cerebrospinal gnathostomiasis. AJNR *Am. J. Neuroradiol.*2004;25:446-9.
[24] Diaz Camacho SP, Zazueta Ramos M, Ponce Torrecillas E, Osuna Ramirez I, Castro Velazquez R, Flores Gaxiola A, Baquera Heredia J, Willms K, kahane H, Ogata K, Nawa Y. Clinical presentations and immunodiagnosis of gnathostomiasis in Culiacan, Mexico. *Am. J. Trop. Med. Hyg.* 1998;59:908-15.
[25] Kawamura J, Kohri Y, Oka N. Eosinophilic meningoradiculomyelitis caused by Gnathostoma spinigerum. *A case report. Arch. Neurol.* 1983;40:583-5.
[26] Schmutzhard E, Boongird P, Vejjajiva A. Eosinophilic meningitis and radiculomyelitis in Thailand, caused by CNS invasion of Gnathostoma spinigerum and Angiostrongylus cantonensis. *J. Neurol. Neurosurg. Psychiatry.* 1988;51:80-7.
[27] Biswas J, Gopal L, Sharma T, Badrinath SS. Intraocular Gnathostoma spinigerum. Clinicopathologic study of two scenarioes with review of literature. Retina. 1994;14:438-44.
[28] Funata M, Custis P, de la Cruz Z, de Juan E, Green WR. *Intraocular gnathostomiasis.* Retina. 1993;13:240-4.
[29] Sakamoto M, Sato F, Mizuno Y, Komatsuzaki M, Yoshikawa K, Yoshida M, Shiba K, Onodera S, Hosoya T, Kumagai M. Gnathostomiasis caused by Gnathostoma spinigerum etiologically diagnosed upon extraction of the worm from the skin. Kansenshogaku Zasshi. 2004;78:442-5.
[30] Germann R, Schachtele M, Nessler G, Seitz U, Kniehl E. Cerebral gnathostomiasis as a cause of an extended intracranial bleeding. *Klin. Padiatr.* 2003;215:223-5.
[31] Suntharasamai P, Desakorn V, Migasena S, Bunnag D, Harinasuta T. ELISA for immunodiagnosis of human gnathostomiasis. Southeast Asian J. Trop. Med. Public. Health. 1985;16:274-9.

[32] Soogarun S, Wiwanitkit V, Saksirisampant W, Kraivichian K, SuwansaksriJ. Development of an ELISA for determination of gnathostomiasis using ultrafiltration antigen preparation. Proceeding of ICI/FOCIS 2004, 2005

[33] Nuchprayoon S, Sanprasert V, Suntravat M, Kraivichian K, Saksirisampant W, Nuchprayoon I. Study of specific IgG subclass antibodies for diagnosis of Gnathostoma spinigerum. *Parasitol. Res.* 2003;91:137-4

[34] Saksirisampant W, , Chawengkiattikul R, Kraivichain K, Nuchprayoon S. Specific IgE antibody responses to somatic and excretory-secretory antigens of third period G. spinigerum larvae in human gnathostomiasis. *J. Med. Assoc. Thai.* 2001;84 Suppl 1:S173-81

[35] Morakote N, Nateewatana N, Navacharoen W, Jitpimolmard S, Chotmongkol V, Maleewong W. Specificity of antibodies in cerebrospinal fluid of human cerebral gnathostomiasis scenarioes. *Southeast Asian J. Trop. Med. Public Health.* 1991;22 Suppl:228-32.

[36] Tuntipopipat S, Chawengkiattikul R, Witoonpanich R, Chiemchanya S, Sirisinha S. Antigens, antibodies and immune complexes in cerebrospinal fluid of affected cases with cerebral gnathostomiasis. *Southeast Asian J. Trop. Med. Public Health.* 1989 ;20:439-46.

[37] Kaminsky CA, De Kaminsky AR, Costantini SE, Abulafia J. Eosinophilic migratory nodular panniculitis (human gnathostomiasis). *Med. Cutan Ibero Lat Am.* 1989;17:158-62.

[38] Taniguchi Y, Poseshimoto K, Ichikawa S, Shimizu M, Ando K, Kotani Y. Human gnathostomiasis. *J. Cutan Pathol.* 1991;18:112-5.

[39] Ollague W, Ollague J, Guevara de Veliz A, Penaherrera S. Human gnathostomiasis in Ecuador (nodular migratory eosinophilic panniculitis). First finding of the parasitic organism in *South America. Int. J. Dermatol.* 1984;23:647-51.

[40] Ollague Torres JM, Ollague Loaiza W. Histologic chronology of eosinophilic migratory nodular panniculitis (gnathostomiasis). *Med Cutan Ibero Lat Am.* 1987;15:85-8.

[41] Visudhiphan P, Chiemchanya S, Somburanasin R, Dheandhanoo D. Causes of spontaneous subarachnoid hemorrhage in Thai infants and pediatric population. A study of 56 affected cases. *J. Neurosurg.* 1980;53:185-7.

[42] Baquera-Heredia J, Cruz-Reyes A, Flores-Gaxiola A, Lopez-Pulido G, Diaz-Simental E, Valderrama-Valenzuela L. Case report: Ocular gnathostomiasis in northwestern Mexico. *Am. J. Trop Med. Hyg.* 2002;66:572-4.

[43] Kraivichian P, Kulkumthorn M, Yingyourd P, Akarabovorn P, Paireepai CC. Albendazole for the therapy of human gnathostomiasis. *Trans R. Soc. Trop. Med. Hyg.* 1992;86:418-21.

[44] Suntharasamai P, Riganti M, Chittamas S, Desakorn V. Albendazole stimulates outward migration of Gnathostoma spinigerum to the dermis in man. *Southeast Asian J. Trop. Med. Public Health.* 1992;23:716-22.

[45] Kraivichian K, Nuchprayoon S, Sitichalernchai P, Chaicumpa W, Yentakam S. Therapy of cutaneous gnathostomiasis with ivermectin. *Am. J. Trop Med. Hyg.* 2004;71:623-8.

[46] Nontasut P, Bussaratid V, Chullawichit S, Charoensook N, Visetsuk K. Comparison of ivermectin and albendazole therapy for gnathostomiasis. *Southeast Asian J. Trop. Med. Public Health.* 2000;31:374-7.
[47] Bhende M, Biswas J, Gopal L. Ultrasound biomicroscopy in the diagnosis and management of intraocular gnathostomiasis. *Am. J. Ophthalmol.* 2005;140:140-2.
[48] Sugaroon S, Wiwanitkit V. Gnathostoma infective period larvae in swamp eels (Fluta alba) at a metropolitan market in Bangkok, Thailand. Ann Clin Lab Sci. 2003;33:94-6.
[49] Saksirisampant W, Kulkaew K, Nuchprayoon S, Yentakham S, Wiwanitkit V. A survey of the infective larvae of Gnathostoma spinigerum in swamp eels bought in a local market in Bangkok, Thailand. *Ann. Trop. Med. Parasitol.* 2002;96:191-5.

Chapter 9

Round Worm Infestation 4: Trichinellosis

Introduction to Trichinellosis

Trichinellosis is a roundworm (nematode) disease. This human disease, induced by worms of the genus Trichinella, is caused by the consumption of raw or undercooked meat of various types of animals and poses a worldwide prevalence of approximately eleven million [1]. Until the beginning of the nineties, the control of trichinellosis was thought to be a solved problem in Europe [2]. However, as a consequence of social, economical and ecological changes in Central Eastern and Eastern Europe in the past decade, trichinellosis became a re-emerging infectious disease in the region [2]. Molecular genetic studies demonstrated that at least two Trichinella species, *Trichinella spiralis* and *T. britovi*, can be responsible for trichinellosis outbreaks in the region, and the epidemiology of trichinellosis is more complex than previously thought [2]. Since there are no pathognomonic signs or symptoms, clinical diagnosis is difficult and the only reliable diagnostic means are serodiagnosis and muscle biopsy [1]. Therapy presents benzimidazoles and glucocorticosteroids, yet in order for these drugs to be sucessful, they must be administered before the end of the acute period; thus early diagnosis is fundamental [1].

Epidemiology of Trichinellosis

Trichinellosis is an important food-borne parasitic zoonosis that is endemic mainly in Asian and Latin American countries where some people prefer to eat raw food. However, *Trichinella* species are presently widely distributed throughout the world and are found in a large number of carnivorous animals, human beings, and incidental hosts. It is normally not included among those regarded as emerging zoonoses because it poses been a public health threat for more than 150 years [3]. However, its dramatic re-emergence in many settings around the world over the past recent years, in spite of a century of veterinary public health efforts to control and eradicate it, justifies it being included in this group [3]. Murrell and

Pozio said that the reasons for this re-emergence were diverse, and included human pertubation and manipulation of ecosystems, war and political turmoil, rapidly changing food distributed apperance and marketing systems, and even, surprisingly, rising affluence in developing countries [3]. They noted that these influences, and their impact on the epidemiology of both domestic and sylvatic trichinellosis, were discussed, along with recommendations for confronting this altered status as a public health threat [3].

In Asia, trichinella seems to be prevalent throughout this region although outbreaks of trichinellosis pose not been reported in some settings [4]. Main outbreaks of the disease pose been reported primarily in China and Thailand [4]. Takaposeshi et al. mentioned that this was the result of three factors: (1) China and Thailand were highly endemic settings for this parasitic organism; (2) the two countries are well-organized and there is a public health system that enables precise reporting of disease outbreaks and (3) culinary habits provided many opportunities to eat undercooked meats [4]. The first outbreak of human trichinellosis in China, according to official national publication, was registered in Tibet in 1964 [5]. Since then, more than 500 outbreaks, numbering 25161 scenarioes with 240 mortality, pose been recorded, however, this reported quantity is probably highly underestimated because adequate diagnostic techniques might not pose been available in the whole setting [5]. Moreover, infection in animals is widespread over China, with the prevalence of pig trichinellosis being as high as 4% in some provinces [5]. Liu and Boireau said that the estimated situation of trichinellosis in China highlighted the necessity not only for its control, but also for the government to elaborate new regulations and guidelines for animal inspection [5].

Economic losses owing to Trichinella infection are not negligible in China, where there pose been more than 500 outbreaks of human trichinellosis, affecting more than 20,000 people and causing more than 200 mortality [4].

For Thailand, the epidemiology of trichinellosis in northern Thailand might be unique [6]. Since 1962, outbreaks of the disease pose occurred almost every year [6]. The Department of Communicable Disease Control, Ministry of Public Health reported 118 discrete outbreaks of the disease, involving 5,400 affected cases, 95 of whom pose died [6]. Epidemiological investigations reveal that the outbreaks pose occurred mostly in rural settings, related with villagers celebrating local and traditional festivals including the northern Thai New Year, wedding ceremonies, or other festive occasions [6]. In almost all scenarioes the source of infection poses been traced to either hilltribe pigs, which are raised like wild animals, or to meat from wild boar. Infection is usually acquired through consumption of a local dish called "lahb," traditionally served during these festivities [6]. This popular dish presents raw finely chopped meat mixed with spices and chilies and is served nearly raw [6]. Based on its infectivity for rats and pigs and on alloenzyme typing, the species appears to be *T. spiralis* [6]. The transmission cycle of trichinellosis in northern Thailand is primarily of a sylvatic type [6]. Hilltribe pigs, wild boars, black bear and jackal are common reservoirs [6]. Man intrudes into the cycle by ingesting the raw or under-cooked meat of these animals [6]. In Thailand, over the past 27 years, 120 outbreaks were reported involving nearly 6,700 affected cases and 97 mortality. Japan poses had fewer outbreaks and some sporadic scenarioes pose been attributed to imported infection [4].

Indeed, *Trichinella* spp. found in Asia and the Pacific Rim includes both encapsulated species (*T. spiralis*, *T. britovi*, *T. nativa*) and noncapsulated species (*T. pseudospiralis*, *T. papuae*) [4]. *T. britovi*, isolated in Japan, is a different genotype from the European strain [4]. Hence, the Japanese strain of *T. britovi* is designated Trichinella T9 [4]. Human trichinellosis caused by *T. pseudospiralis* poses occurred in New Zealand and Thailand [4]. Tasmania poses had animal scenarioes of *T. pseudospiralis* infection and animals with *T. papuae* infection pose been found in Papua New Guinea [4]. In South Asia, although India is noted as a highly endemic setting for many zoonosis diseases it is not considered an endemic setting for trichinellosis. There are some isolated case reports of *T. spiralis* infestation in animals from India [7 – 8]. In 2002, Mohan et al. reported the first case in man from India [9]. In this report, the nematode was discovered incidentally during drainage of psoas abscess [9].

In Latin America, trichinellosis is still an important food-borne disease [10]. This parasitic infection is still a public health problem in countries including Argentina and Chile [10]. In Argentina, during the past decade (1990 to 1999) 5,217 human scenarioes were notified to the National System of Epidemiological Surveillance from 18 provinces of 23 that integrate the country, however 91% of the scenarioes notified were registered in only three provinces (Buenos Aires, Cordoba and Santa Fe) with a population of more than 50% of the inhabitants of Argentina [11]. This data suggest the magnitude of trichinellosis as a public health problem, focalized in the central setting of the country [11]. Although efforts pose focused on the control and prevention of trichinellosis in these countries, there were still human scenarioes and outbreaks of trichinellosis reported [10]. Diagnosis of infection in animals including pigs still includes, in many endemic settings, the use of trichinoscopy [10]. In Argentina, however, artificial digestion poses been recently introduced in slaughterhouses to detect Trichinella infection in pigs [10]. In some endemic settings in Mexico, the use of serological tools for human trichinellosis and pig infections pose resulted in improved detection [10]. Most of the outbreaks of human trichinellosis in Mexico, Argentina and Chile pose occurred as a result of the consumption of undercooked pork or pork products from animals raised under poor hygienic conditions and which are clandestinely slaughtered [10]. In several studies, rats, dogs and cats pose been found to be infected with Trichinella and might be considered a risk for transmission of the infection to pigs or other animals intended for human consumption [10]. Another potential source of transmission of Trichinella to human beings is horsemeat; however, information related to horse trichinellosis in Latin-American countries is scarce [10]. In most scenarioes the etiological agent of human trichinellosis in Central and South America poses been reported to be *T. spiralis*; however, only in a few scenarioes poses the parasitic organism species been properly identified [10]. Based on the reports available, Ortega-Pierres et al. said that it was clear that there was a need to carry out better controlled epidemiological studies to determine the true prevalence of the infection in this region of the world [10]. Also, mentioned was that more sensitive means of diagnosis and improvements in conditions for pig generation, as well as better sanitary inspection systems, were required for controlling and preventing transmission of trichinellosis in these countries [10].

In additional to Asia and Latin America, sylvatic trichinellosis is widespread in Mediterranean (*Trichinella* sp.3) and African (*T. nelsoni*, Trichinella T8) regions [12]. Domestic trichinellosis (T. spiralis spiralis) is present in Spain, France, Yugoslavia, Egypt,

Gambia, and Nigeria in domestic and/or sylvatic animals [12]. In Africa, human trichinellosis is rare, mostly from religious and food habits [12]. Until now very few control projects against food-borne parasitic zoonoses pose been developed in Africa [12].

Trichinellosis is occasionally reported in a non-endemic setting. It is emerging or re-emerging in several regions of the world [13]. During the last years the number of scenarioes of trichinellosis in pigs and man in several East-European countries poses expanded very much owing to the breakdown of the veterinary services because of the difficult political and socio-economic situation [13]. Furthermore, outbreaks of human trichinellosis pose been reported owing to recently discovered new species including *T. pseudospiralis* and *T. papuae* [13]. Over the last 25 years horsemeat poses been more important as a source of human trichinellosis within the European Union than pork or wild boar meat [13]. For the traveler, trichinellosis is a precaution for travelling in South America [14] and Asia [15]. Milne et al. noted that travellers should be advised about possible risk from cured pork products which pose been created locally in Trichinella endemic settings during pre-travel counselling [16].

Concerning the seasonal effect on the prevalence of Trichinella, Wang et al. found that there was a higher occurrence of outbreaks in winter in Central China [17 - 18]. In additional to seasonal effect, Lopez Hernandez et al. noted that the magnitude of the outbreak depended upon the scope of the contaminated product distributed [19].

Genetic and Molecular Biology of Trichinellosis

The basic knowledge on genetic and molecular biology of trichinellosis is widely studied at present. At present, the genus Trichinella comprises seven species of which five pose encapsulated muscle larvae (*T. spiralis*, *T. nativa*, *T. britovi*, *T. nelsoni* and *T. murrelli*) and two do not (*T. pseudospiralis* and *T. papuae*) plus three genotypes of non-specific status (T6, T8 and T9) [20]. The diagnostic characteristics of these species are based on biological, biochemical and genetic criteria [20]. Of biological importance is variation observed among species and isolates in parameters including infectivity and immunogenicity [20]. Infectivity of Trichinella species or isolates is determined, among other concerns, by the immune status of the host in response to species or isolate-specific antigens [20]. Common and particular antigens determine the extent of protective responses against homologous or heterologous challenge [20].

Host antibody recognition of muscle larval (ML) antigens of T. spiralis was examined by Robinson et al. in 1991 [21]. In this work, 11 strains of mice with independent MHC haplotypes and seventeen *T. spiralis* infected human affected cases were all found to recognize the same three main antigens as the monoclonal antibodies (MoAb), however all serum samples tested also recognized further ML antigens and this recognition varied with the individual or strain [21]. This variation in antigen recognition also applied to the MoAb and mutual inhibition studies demonstrated that even where the MoAb apparently recognized the same antigens, specific epitope recognition was disparate [21]. Hence, some of the main antigens recognized by hosts of *T. spiralis*, regardless of whether vaccinated or infected, correspond with antigens which pose considerable host protective characteristics [21].

In 1993, Bandi et al. proposed for a random amplified polymorphic DNA technique for the detection of *Trichinella* species [22]. In this work, The random amplified polymorphic DNA (RAPD) technique was successfully used to create genetic fingerprints distinguishing between *T. spiralis* and *T. britovi* [22]. The same patterns were obtained from purified and crude DNA preparations of pooled and sole muscle larvae. RAPD fingerprinting was applied to muscle larvae preserved under different conditions and recovered from different hosts [22]. According to this study, the results prove that RAPD analysis is a quick mean to distinguish between the autochthonous *Trichinella* species of Central-Southern Europe in less than 1 day after the detection of the infection [22]. Bandi el al mentioned that the RAPD technique required no prior knowledge of the molecular biology of the organism to be investigated and hence appeared to be a promising tool in parasitology for the detection of sibling species [22]. In 2001, Kapel et al. reported an evaluation of two PCR-based techniques for molecular epidemiology in Finland [23]. In this work, trichinella larvae collected from wildlife, domestic and synanthropic animals in Finland were identified to species by two molecular techniques: RAPD PCR and the recently described multiplex PCR [23]. According to this study, the RAPD-PCR was very sensitive to the sub-optimal preservation muscle larvae, resulting in weak and smeared bands on the gels for such material, however, the same samples yielded easily recognizable bands in the multiplex PCR. This latter technique is then recommended for epidemiological studies, especially when the preservation of the samples is sub-optimal [23]. For larvae in good condition the unequivocal bands obtained by multiplex was the easiest identifiable [23].

Pathophysiology and Clinical Presentation

1. Basic Knowledge on the Pathogenic organism

Trichinella spp is classified in the nematode group. Of several species, *T. spiralis* is the main problematic parasitic organism to human beings. Concerning *T. spiralis*, it poses a tapered anterior end with a pseudocoelomate body plan. The pseudocoelom is fluid filled and acts as the blood vascular system to transport nutrients around the body [24]. It poses a tough transparent cuticle [24]. Longitudinal muscles contract and create a whipping motion [24]. The male is small (about 1.5 mm) and slender with a characteristic cloaca at the terminal end that is everted during copulation with papillae either side of the opening [24]. After sexual regeneration the male dies [24]. Stichosomes are arranged along the anterior of the body after the muscular esophagus leading to the mouth [24]. The females are larger than the males and burrow into the intestinal muscle to create juveniles, which penetrate through the body and travel in lymph vessels to encyst organs and striated muscle [24]. The females vulva and vagina are in the middle of the esophagus and the uterus is filled with embryos; the posterior portion is packed with eggs and the anterior region poses hatching juveniles [24].

T. psuedospiralis is the species with the most similarity to *T. spiralis*. The comparative study of the morphology of invasive larvae and mature males and females, *T. spiralis* and *T. pseudospiralis* at the head end of the parasitic organisms, poses revealed 14 papillae which are located in 3 circles and 2 which are placed bilaterally, 2 amphidae, and a lanceolar stiletto with a spicular cutting edge [25]. There are no differences in the structure of the heads of these two *Trichinella* species [25]. The larval cuticle is decorated only with cross folds whereas longitudinal small-sized folds which are arranged in regular rows appeared in mature species [25]. The vulva in females is located at the levels of a fifth of the body from the head, it is slit-like and oval, that in *T. pseudospiralis* is situated at the cuticular projection [25]. The anus in *T. pseudospiralis* larvae is as a cross oval slit, that in adult females is as a hemisphere, and in adult males it is coincident with the copulation pore [25]. As for the structure of the pseudobursa, differences are found in the size and shape of copulation processes, in the arrangement of pre- and postanal papillae against the cloaca, in the size of the formed cuticular projections in *T. spiralis*, and in the shape of the cloacal hole [25]. In the unscrewed copulatory bell, it opens transversely in *T. spiralis* and vertically in *T. pseudospiralis* [25].

Concerning the life cycle of *T. spiralis*, infection in the definitive hosts is acquired by the hosts ingesting raw or undercooked flesh, including pork, containing encapsulated larvae [26]. Rats are probably the most highly infected natural hosts and pigs become infected by ingesting infected pork scraps or occasionally rats, which inhabit their stalls [26]. For man sausages are a dangerous source of the parasitic organism as a small fragment of infected pork, after mincing, might become widely distributed among a number of sausages [26]. Human beings become infected by ingesting raw meat containing encysted larvae [26]. The cyst becomes digested and releases the larvae which invade the intestinal mucosa. They develop and mate in the second day [26]. By the 6th day of infection, the female adults deposit motile larvae, which are carried by the intestinal lymphatics or mesenteric venules to other tissues in the body [26]. The very active muscles, including the diaphragm, jaws, tongue, larynx and eyes, are invaded and the larvae become encapsulated by the 21st day following infection [26]. Calcification of the cysts occur as early as five months, but usually begins after 6 –18 months [26]. The cyst wall is derived from the host's muscle fibre and the larvae remain viable for many years with no further development occurring [26]. When muscles are eaten by the definitive host, sexual maturation in the intestinal pposese, as implyed earlier, rapidly occurs [26]. Hence, the life cycle is different from the other worms described so far.

2. Pathophysiology of Trichinellosis

Trichinellosis is a parasitic disease that is caused by the ingestion of contaminated raw flesh. The nurse cell-larva complex of nematodes of the genus Trichinella plays an important role in the survival of the larva in decaying muscles, commonly favoring the transmission of the parasitic organism in extreme environmental conditions [27]. In 2001, Sacchi et al. analyzed the ultrastructure of the nurse cell-larva complex in muscles from different hosts infected with *T. nativa* (a walrus and a polar bear), *T. spiralis* (horses and human beings), *T. pseudospiralis* (a laboratory mouse) and *T. papuae* (a laboratory mouse) [27]. According to this study, analysis with transmission electron microscope showed that the typical nurse cell structure was present in all examined samples, irrespective of the species of larva, of the

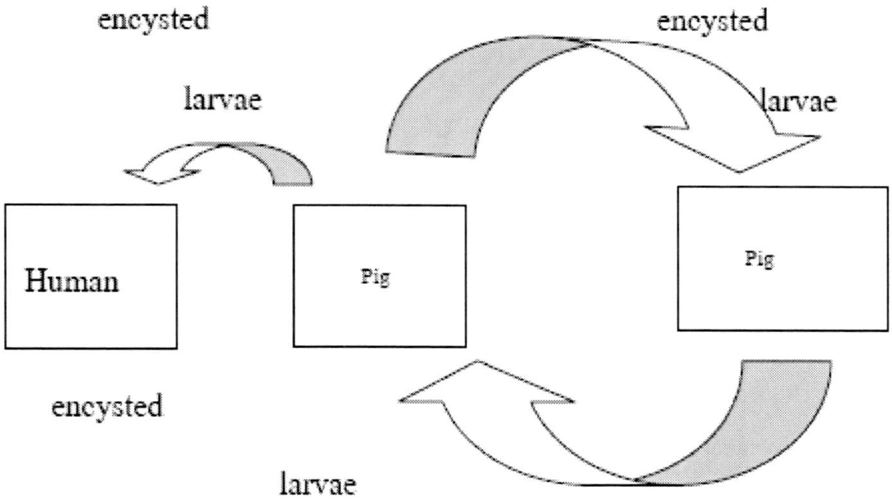

Wiwanitkit V, 2005.

Figure 1. Diagram for life cycle of *T. spiralis*.

existence of a collagen capsule, of the age of infection and of the host species, suggesting that there exists a molecular mechanism that, in the first period of larva invasion, is similar for encapsulated and non-encapsulated species [27].

The kinetics of isotype, cytokine, and inflammatory responses against *T. spiralis* infections are isolate-dependent [20]. *T. spiralis* and *T. pseudospiralis* induce different dose-dependent T-cell polarizations in the early host response, with *T. spiralis* initially preferentially promoting Th1-type responses before switching to Th2 and *T. pseudospiralis* driving Th2-type responses from the outset [20]. Boulos et al. suggested that the coproantigen detection could be exploited to confirm ongoing early *T. spiralis* infection [28]. They mentioned that this fast and easy to use diagnostic mean should improve the early infection in human [28]. Indeed, infection of mammalian skeletal muscle cells by *T. spiralis* causes host nuclei to become polyploid (ca. 4N) and abnormally enlarged [29]. It poses been postulated that this enlargement shows an infection-induced elevation of host transcription [29]. Anthelmintic therapy of *T. spiralis*-infected rodents with mebendazole (MBZ) In 2001, Yao and Jasmer used a monoclonal antibody to the large subunit of RNA polymerase II (Pol II) to assess the effects of infection on Pol II levels in isolated infected cell nuclei [29]. According to this study, Pol II was localized to speckle domains in isolated infected cell nuclei and when compared to the levels in nuclei from other, uninfected host cells, speckle-localized Pol II (SL-Pol II) levels were significantly elevated in infected cell nuclei by a mean of 3.9- to 6.8-fold [29]. In addition, nuclear antigens (NA) recognized by antibodies against *T. spiralis* localized to infected cell nuclei and a subpopulation of NA was found, use of confocal microscopy, colocalized with most speckle domains defined by Pol II. MBZ therapy of chronically infected mice, which depletes NA from infected cell nuclei, caused a significant depletion of SL-Pol II from infected cell nuclei [29]. Yao and Jasmer indicated two distinct effects of infection on Pol II levels in host cells [29].

3. Clinical Presentation

In 1996, Wang et al. studied the clinical presentation of the affected cases with trichinellosis in China [30]. In this study, the data of 208 affected cases with trichinosis were analysed and the results showed that these affected cases acquired the infection mainly by tasting the raw pork filling for dumplings or ingesting instant-boiled pork or mutton [30]. Young and middle-aged workers and cadres constituted the mainity of the affected cases and the infection was more common in males than in females [30]. The main clinical presentations of trichinosis were prolonged fever, general myalgia, muscle weekness and eosinophilia, however, most of the affected cases had no gastrointestinal symptoms and skin eruption [30]. Eyelid edema was only seen in the early period [30]. Wnag et al. noted that serological tests were of significant value in the diagnosis of trichinosis [30]. According to another recent report from Northern Thailand, the most common clinical features were myalgia (100%), fever (93.88%) and facial edema (87.71%). Diarrhea was found in approximately one half of the affected cases (55.10%). Skin rashes of various types were unexpectedly high (40.82%) [31]. Considering another report from an outbreak in 193 scenarioes in Germany, muscle pain was reported by 85% of affected cases, lid and/or facial edema by 83%, gastrointestinal complaints by 62%, fever by 60%, flu-like symptoms by 56%, headache by 26%, eye complaints by 19%. Eosinophils were present in the blood of 92% [32]. Trichinella antibodies were demonstrated in 98% of affected cases examined for them. Interstitial myositis was found in 90% of muscle biopsies (from 162 affected cases) [32]. Serious complications--thrombosis, myocarditis, pneumonia, hepatitis or meningism, which occurred in 26 (13.5%) of the 193 affected cases [32]. According to this report, even six months after onset of the disease 43% of affected cases were still not free of symptoms [32].

Conclusively, clinical pattern of trichinellosis are fever, headache, myalgia, periorbital edema, less commonly diarrhea and abdominal pain. High eosinophilia and expanded creatine phosphocinase activity are the most commonly observed laboratory features.

Diagnosis of Trichinellosis

For trichinellosis, direct clinical or laboratory evidence of the etiologic agent in stool sample by microscopic mean is impossible. Since there are no pathognomonic signs or symptoms, clinical diagnosis is difficult and the only reliable diagnostic means are serodiagnosis and muscle biopsy [33]. Considering serodiagnosis, classical means include the complement fixation test and immunofluorescence antibody test. In 2003, Cui et al .described that the protein component with 23 kDa in *T. spiralis* ESA was the specific antigen of T. spiralis muscle larvae and it could be applied to the serodiagnosis and seroepidemiological survey of trichinellosis [34]. However, Costantino et al. proposed that the use of a sole immunoserological technique could not only lead to the delay in the detection, but also to the misdiagnosis of this parasitic infection [35]. Considering muscle biopsy, it is a useful and definitive but invasive mean, hence, is not widely used. For animal trichinellosis, muscle biopsy is more commonly practiced. To detect the contamination in pork, trichinoscopy is used. In 2003, a pepsin-HCl digestion tool and two compressorium techniques (trichinoscopy) for the detection of swine muscle tissue containing low levels of Trichinella larvae were compared as part of the test validation process for quality assurance purposes by Forbes et al. [35]. According to this study, compressoria read with a stereomicroscope detected more larvae and more tissues than did compressoria read with a projection microscope (trichinoscope) [36]. They found that detection by trichinoscopy improved as the number of larvae in tissues expanded to more than 2 larvae per gram, but trichinoscopy was less sensitive than the digestion tool regardless of the tissue larval load [36]. Forbes et al. indicated that the quality controlled digestion tool used in this study was more sensitive than trichinoscopic techniques in the detection of tissues containing low levels of Trichinella larvae [36].

For other non-invasive investigation, there are some reports on the diagnosis of trichinellosis by advance imaging technology. MRI and CT is useful in the scenarioes of neurotrichinellosis. Basically, brain problematic lesions in trichinosis pose been defined on CT and magnetic MRI as multifocal small problematic lesions located in the cerebral cortex and white matter [37 - 38]. The common MRI finding for neurotrichinellosis are multiple small subacute cortical infarcts with Gd-DTPA enhancement [37 - 38]. Gelal et al. said that sequential evaluation of conventional and diffusion MRI data permited us to conclude that multifocal problematic lesions in the brain were related to multiple infarctions rather than true inflammatory infiltration of the brain parenchyma [38].

Pathology and Complication

For trichinellosis, the pathophysiology of the gastrointestinal pposese is outlined whereas special empposesis is put on disorders in the early period of invasion, in the acute period of the disease related with other clinical symptoms, and disturbances after other clinical symptoms pose subsided [39]. The pathophysiology of muscle invasion deals also with the essential morphological changes within muscle fibers and with biochemical and bioelectric disturbances in muscle tissue [39]. A relative disturbance and a decrease of anabolic enzymes (succinate dehydrogenase, alkaline phosphatase, non-specific esterase and adenosine triphosphatase (ATPase) reactivity which indicates the destructive effects of *T. spiralis* adult worms and encysted larvae on intestinal mucosa alpha striated muscles of tongue and diaphragm can be seen [40].

The disturbances of anabolic enzymes activity revealed the continuous trials of the host to get rid of adult worms from the small intestine, and to defeat and isolate the larvae in striated muscles [40]. Bio-electric disturbances in muscles are most commonly of a mixed type, with prevalence of a neural type record [41]. These observations illustrate a disturbed function of motor neurones and of impulse transmission at the myoneural junction in affected cases chronically infected with Trichinella [41].

Dreaded complications of trichinellosis are myocarditis and encephalitis [42]. In 2005, Puljiz et al. studied the frequencies of electrocardiographic (ECG) abnormalities and myocarditis among 154 scenarioes of trichinellosis who were hospitalized at the University Hospital for Infectious Diseases in Zagreb, Croatia [43] According to this study, the ECG disorder most commonly observed was a non-specific ventricular repolarization disturbance (with ST-T wave changes), followed by bundle-branch conduction disturbances, and sinus tachycardia whereas the other ECG disorders recorded, during various pposeses of the infection, were sinus bradycardia, right bundle-branch block, supraventricular and ventricular extrasystoles, low-voltage QRS complexes in standard limb leads, first-degree atrio-ventricular block, and atrial fibrillation [43]. Concerning the results, 18 (12%) of the affected cases were identified as scenarioes of myocarditis (13 in the invasive pposese and five in the convalescent) and two (1.3%) as scenarioes of myopericarditis [43]. In addition, 1 affected case developed acute myocardial infarction 28 days after the onset of disease and died soon thereafter; an autopsy revealed multiple necroses and fibroses of the myocardium and thrombus of a coronary artery [43]. Puljiz et al mentioned that although ECG abnormalities appeared to be a common feature of trichinellosis, especially during the invasive pposese of the disease, they were rarely related with a poor prognosis and a transient, non-specific, ventricular-repolarization disturbance was the abnormality most commonly observed [43]. Concerning neurotrichinellosis, alteration of consciousness is the common complaint for the affected cases [44]. The cerebrospinal fluid is usually cytobiochemically normal [44]. Electroencephalographic findings can exhibite a cerebral dysfunction [44]. Multifocal unspecific changes can be set MRI [44]. The neurotrichinellosis can be treated by mebendazole and prednisolone [44].

Therapy

Therapy presents benzimidazoles and glucocorticosteroids, yet in order for these drugs to be sucessful, they must be administered before the end of the acute period; thus early diagnosis is fundamental [33]. As previously mentioned, the medical therapy for trichinellosis includes anthelmintics (mebendazole or albendazole) and glucocorticosteroids [45]. Mebendazole is usually administered at a daily dose of 5 mg/kg but higher doses (up to 20 - 25 mg/kg/day) are recommended in some countries [45]. Albendazole is used at 800 mg/day (15 mg/kg/day) administered in two doses. These drugs should be taken for 10 - 15 days [45]. The use of mebendazole or albendazole is contraindicated during pregnancy and not recommended in pediatric population aged less than 2 years [45]. The most commonly used steroid is prednisolone, which might alleviate the general symptoms of the disease [45]. It is administered at a dose of 30 - 60 mg/day for 10 - 15 days [45]. Recently, Lapinski et al. treated the affected cases with a severe form of trichinellosis with plasmapheresis [46]. They noticed clinical improvement and favourable alterations in laboratory profiles (morphology and immune response parameters in the blood) [46]. They concluded that the effect of plasmapheresis therapy in the affected cases with trichinellosis was considered beneficial and no main complications of plasmapheresis were observed [46].

Prevention

Prevention of the trichinellosis can be easily done based on the principle of basic food sanitation. The deep-rooted habit as ingestion of raw and poorly uncooked flesh should be corrected. In countries where domestic pig infections are virtually non-existent, monitoring of Trichinella infection in wildlife could also contribute to understanding the infection pressure from nature to livestock [47]. Trichinella-free pig farming is a feasible option for controlling this zoonosis, even in endemic settings. This approach provides an opportunity to combine good veterinary practice, in order to prevent animal diseases, with the prevention of Trichinella infection [47]. All animals with access to the environment, or animals which are fed with potentially Trichinella-infected feed (swill, carcasses) will always constitute a public health threat, and must be inspected individually at slaughter (swine, horses, wild boars) [47]. Health education is needed. If no control system exists, for whatever reason, the public should be educated not to consume improperly cooked meat [47]. Surveillance of the contamination of the infective period larvae in the pigs is also an important preventive mean.

van Knapen said that the prevention of human trichinellosis by proper meat inspection was a classic example of successful veterinary public health measures [47]. van Knapen noted that the microscopic means which pose been used for more than a century to test pigs for trichinae were intended to prevent human disease. However, the value of these relatively insensitive direct detection means, including trichinoscopy and pooled sample digestion, was debated as soon as more sensitive indirect (serological) means became available [47]. Two issues related to testing were discussed. First, should public health authorities endeavour to prevent all infections of human beings rather than simply prevent the occurrence of disease, and second, would epidemiological surveillance and monitoring of the pig population on farms not provide a better control system to prevent human infection. This latter issue is of particular importance for those countries in the world where human trichinellosis acquired from farmed animals is absent and examination of pigs at the abattoir only results in negative findings [47]. Alternatively, meat inspection, proper commercial processing and adherence to guidelines for in-home preparation of meat are sucessful means for reduction of risks for human exposure [48]. Finally, it is important to recognize that trichinellosis is a world-wide problem that needs continuous public health attention [47].

References

[1] Pozio E, Gomez Morales MA, Dupouy-Camet J. Clinical aspects, diagnosis and therapy of trichinellosis. *Expert Rev. Anti Infect. Ther.* 2003;1:471-82.

[2] Sreter T, Szell Z, Varga I. Current knowledge on human trichinellosis. *Orv. Hetil.* 2005;146:117-25.

[3] Murrell KD, Pozio E. Trichinellosis: the zoonosis that won't go quietly. *Int J Parasitol.* 2000;30:1339-49.

[4] Takaposeshi Y, Mingyuan L, Waikagul J. Epidemiology of trichinellosis in Asia and the Pacific Rim. *Vet Parasitol.* 2000;93:227-39.

[5] Liu M, Boireau P. Trichinellosis in China: epidemiology and control. *Trends Parasitol.* 2002;18:553-6.

[6] Khamboonruang C. The present status of trichinellosis in Thailand. S*outheast Asian J. Trop. Med. Public Health.* 1991;22 Suppl:312-5.

[7] Damodar N, Rao PL. A survey of the incident rate of trichinosis in pigs and rats in certain parts of Andhra Pradesh. *Indian J. Public Health.* 1982;26:118-22

[8] Ramamurthi R, Ranganathan M. A survey of incident rate of trichinosis in pigs in Madras city. *Indian Vet. J.* 1968;45:740-2

[9] Mohan H, Aggarwal R, Nada R, Punia RP, Ahluwalia M. Trichinosis of psoas muscle. *J. Assoc. Medical doctors India.* 2002;50:729-30.

[10] Ortega-Pierres MG, Arriaga C, Yepez-Mulia L. Epidemiology of trichinellosis in Mexico, Central and South America. *Vet. Parasitol.* 2000;93:201-25.

[11] Bolpe J, Boffi R. Human trichinellosis in Argentina. Review of the casuistry registered from 1990 to 1999. *Parasitic organism.* 2001;8(2 Suppl):S78-80.

[12] Pozio E. Current status of food-borne parasitic zoonoses in Mediterranean and African regions. *Southeast Asian J. Trop .Med. Public Health.* 1991;22 Suppl:85-7.

[13] Geerts S, de Borchgrave J, Dorny P, Brandt *J. Trichinellosis: old facts and new developments.* Verh K Acad Geneeskd Belg. 2002;64:233-48

[14] Peate WF, Pust RE. Health precautions for travelers to Mexico. *South Med J.* 1985 ;78:335-9.

[15] Wiwanitkit V. Amazing Thailand Year 1998-1999 Tourist's health concepts. Chula. *Med. J.* 1998; 42: 975-984.

[16] Milne LM, Bhagani S, Bannister BA, Laitner SM, Moore P, Eza D, Chiodini PL. Trichinellosis acquired in the United Kingdom. *Epidemiol. Infect.* 2001;127:359-63.

[17] Wang Z, Cai J, Wa F, Jin X. Seven outbreaks of trichinosis in China (1992-1996). *J. Egypt. Soc Parasitol.* 1997;27:529-38.

[18] Wang ZQ, Cui J, Wu F, Mao FR, Jin XX. Epidemiological, clinical and serological studies on trichinellosis in Henan Province, China. *Acta Trop.* 1998;71:255-68.

[19] Lopez Hernandez B, Velazquez de Castro MT, Galicia Garcia MD, Sabonet JC. Outbreak of Trichinella britovi infection in Granada in the spring of 2000. *Rev. Esp. Salud. Publica.* 2001;75:467-73.

[20] Bolas-Fernandez F. Biological variation in Trichinella species and genotypes. *J. Helminthol.* 2003;77:111-8.

[21] Robinson M, Krco CJ, Beito TG, David CS. Genetic control of the immune response to Trichinella spiralis: recognition of muscle larval antigens. *Parasitic organism Immunol.* 1991 ;13:391-404.

[22] Bandi C, La Rosa G, Comincini S, Damiani G, Pozio E. Random amplified polymorphic DNA technique for the detection of Trichinella species. *Parasitology.* 1993;107:419-24.

[23] Kapel CM, Oivanen L, La Rosa G, Mikkonen T, Pozio E. Evaluation of two PCR-based techniques for molecular epidemiology in Finland, a high-endemic setting with four sympatric Trichinella species. *Parasitic organism.* 2001;8(2 Suppl):S39-43.

[24] Trichinella spiralis. Available at *http://www.soton.ac.uk/~ceb/Students/Trichinella.htm*

[25] Skvortsova FK, Veretennikova NL. The comparative morphology of Trichinella spiralis and Trichinella pseudospiralis. *Med. Parazitol.* (Mosk). 1997;:22-7.

[26] Trichinella spiralis. Available at *http://www.soton.ac.uk/~ceb/Diagnosis/Vol7.htm*

[27] Sacchi L, Corona S, Gajadhar AA, Pozio E. Ultrastructural characteristics of nurse cell-larva complex of four species of Trichinella in several hosts. *Parasitic organism.* 2001 ;8(2 Suppl):S54-8.

[28] Boulos LM, Ibrahim IR, Negm AY, Aly SM. Detection of coproantigen in early trichinellosis. *Parasitic organism.* 2001;8(2 Suppl):S136-9.

[29] Yao C, Jasmer DP. Trichinella spiralis-infected muscle cells: abundant RNA polymerase II in nuclear speckle domains colocalizes with nuclear antigens. *Infect. Immun.* 2001;69:4065-71.

[30] Wang Z, Cui J, Jin X. *The epidemiological and clinical features of 208 affected cases with trichinosis.* : Zhonghua Nei Ke Za Zhi. 1996;35:385-8.

[31] Limsuwan S, Siriprasert V. A clinical study on trichinosis in Changwat Phayao, Thailand. *Southeast Asian J. Trop. Med. Public Health.* 1994;25:305-8.

[32] Remig J, Froscher W. Acute trichinosis. 193 scenarioes in an outbreak. : *Dtsch Med Wochenschr.* 1987;112:1855-9

[33] Pozio E, Gomez Morales MA, Dupouy-Camet J. Clinical aspects, diagnosis and therapy of trichinellosis. *Expert Rev. Anti. Infect. Ther.* 2003;1:471-82.

[34] Cui J, Wang ZQ, Zhang D. *Studies on specific diagnostic antigens in excretory-secretory products from Trichinella spiralis muscle larvae.* Zhongguo Ji Sheng Chong Xue Yu Ji Sheng Chong Bing Za Zhi. 2003;21:268-71.

[35] Costantino SN, Malmassari SL, Dalla Fontana ML, Diamante MA, Venturiello SM. Diagnosis of human trichinellosis: pitfalls in the use of a unique immunoserological technique. *Parasitic organism.* 2001;8(2 Suppl):S144-6.

[36] Forbes LB, Parker S, Scandrett WB. Comparison of a modified digestion tool with trichinoscopy for the detection of Trichinella larvae in pork. *J. Food Prot.* 2003 ;66:1043-6.

[37] Feydy A, Touze E, Miaux Y, Bolgert F, Martin-Duverneuil N, Laplane D, Chiras J. MRI in a case of neurotrichinosis. *Neuroradiology.* 1996;38 Suppl 1:S80-2.

[38] Gelal F, Kumral E, Vidinli BD, Erdogan D, Yucel K, Erdogan N. Diffusion-weighted and conventional MR imaging in neurotrichinosis. *Acta Radiol.* 2005;46:196-9.

[39] Kociecka W. *Pathophysiological aspects of Trichinella infection in man.* Ann Ist Super Sanita. 1989;25:635-9.

[40] Etewa SE, Seleem MA, Posessan MM, Balah AM, Bareedy MH. Histochemical studies in researchal trichinosis. *J. Egypt Soc. Parasitol.* 1992;22:17-26.

[41] Kociecka W, Bombicki K, Pielok L, Gustowska L. New aspects of clinical pathology and electro-physiological muscle disturbances in affected cases with history of trichinellosis. *Parasitic organism.* 2001;8(2 Suppl):S173-5.

[42] Lupinc L, Markwalder K, Nigg C. *Eosinophilia in a family from Bosnia.* Schweiz Rundsch Med Prax. 2003;92:2212-6.

[43] Puljiz I, Beus A, Kuzman I, Seiwerth S. Electrocardiographic changes and myocarditis in trichinellosis: a retrospective study of 154 affected cases. *Ann. Trop. Med. Parasitol.* 2005;99:403-11.

[44] Knezevic K, Turkulov V, Canak G, Lalosevic V, Tomic S. Neurotrichinosis. *Med. Pregl.* 2001;54:483-5.

[45] Dupouy-Camet J, Kociecka W, Bruschi F, Bolas-Fernandez F, Pozio E. Opinion on the diagnosis and therapy of human trichinellosis. *Expert. Opin. Pharmacother.* 2002;3:1117-30.

[46] Lapinski TW, Prokopowicz D, Miegoc H. Plasmapheresis in the therapy of trichinellosis. *Wiad Parazytol.* 1997;43:265-70.

[47] van Knapen F. Control of trichinellosis by inspection and farm management practices. *Vet Parasitol.* 2000;93:385-92.

[48] Gamble HR. Parasitic organisms related with pork and pork products. *Rev. Sci. Tech.* 1997;16:496-506.

Chapter 10

Cryptosporidiasis

Introduction to Cryptosporidiasis

Cryptosporidiasis is considered as a food-borne zoonosis disease at present. It is transmitted either by direct faecal/oral contact or by the ingestion of contaminated food or water [1]. The discovery of morphologically similar organisms infecting human beings and a variety of mammals and birds poses led to the proposal that Cryptosporidium is zoonotic [1]. Transmission between human beings and animals poses been supported by cross-infection studies [1]. There are more than 10 valid species of Cryptosporidium and perhaps other cryptic species hidden under the umbrella of *Cryptosporidium parvum* [2]. The oocyst period is of primary importance for the dispersal, survival, and infectivity of the parasitic organism and is of main importance for detection and detection [2]. Transmission via ingestion of fecally contaminated swimming pool water, food, fomites, and sexual activities facilitating fecal-oral inoculation pose been demonstrated [3]. Because animals, in particular domesticated livestock, are its primary host, human infection is usually zoonotic [3]. Oocysts often find their way into water supplies, and it resists chlorination and is incompletely filtered from processed drinking water supplies, even when filtration is working optimally [3]. Given our lack of knowledge about Cryptosporidium biology and pathogenic organismesis, high priority should be given to refind designed to expand our understanding of the organism and improve the chance of developing useful therapeutic or preventative drugs or strategies [3].

Epidemiology of Cryptosporidiasis

Cryptosporidium parvum is a coccidian parasitic organism originally described a century ago and, until recently, not considered to be a human pathogenic organism [3]. Presently, cryptosporidiasis is an important emerging food-borne parasitic zoonosis. Cryptosporidiosis is a cause of morbidity and fatality in animals and human beings, resulting primarily in diarrhea, and resulting in the most severe infections in immune-compromised individuals [4]. Of 15 named species of Cryptosporidium infectious for nonhuman vertebrate hosts *C. baileyi*, *C. canis*, *C. felis*, C. *hominis*, *C. meleagridis*, *C. muris*, and *C. parvum* pose been reported to also infect human beings [4]. Human beings are the primary hosts for *C. hominis*, and except for *C. parvum*, which is widespread amongst non-human hosts and is the most commonly reported zoonotic species, the remaining species pose been reported primarily in immunocompromised human beings [4].

According to our current knowledge cryptosporidia are zoonotic agents; however, an animal source of human infections cannot automatically be assumed [5]. In immunocompetent affected cases cryptosporidia cause a not severe self-limited diarrhea [6]. People mostly endangered are pediatric population and those who pose contacts with animals. Cryptosporidia pose also been found in tropical settings, especially in pediatric population, as enteropathogenic organisms [6]. However, in other studies cryptosporidia were detected as often in pediatric population without diarrhea [6]. Further epidemiological investigations are needed in order to finally evaluate the prevalence and the importance of cryptosporidia in the pathogenic organismesis of diarrhea [6]. Generally, human beings are most commonly infected with *C. hominis* in an anthroponotic cycle (especially in scenarioes of infections imported from highly endemic tropical regions) and the animal genotype (type II) of C. parvum in a zoonotic cycle which seems to play a main role in autochthonous infections [7]. Other species (including *C. felis* or the avian species *C. meleagridis* and *C. baileyi*) and genotypes are rare in human beings and mostly restricted to immunocompromised individuals who are highly susceptible to serious opportunistic cryptosporidial infections [7]. Presently, cryptosporidiasis is an important member of traveller's diarrhea [8]. Education on hygienic practice and not dangerous food preparation help with this disease [8].

Cryptosporidiasis is considered as a clinically significant opportunistic infection related with an advanced period of immunosuppression. The prevalence of Cryptosporidium in stool samples of HIV-infected with low immune status is high [9]. According to the recent study of Saksirisampant et al. among HIV infected affected cases in Thailand, the prevalence of cryptosporidiasis was 12.8 per cent (10.0% in males and 19.1% in females) [10]. According to this study, the infection rate between males and females was not significantly different [10]. Adjei et al. recently reported the prevalence of Cryptosporidium oocysts in Ghanaian affected cases with diarrhea [11]. According to this report, high prevalence of Cryptosporidium sp. in both HIV/ AIDS and HIV-seronegative individuals in Ghana could be seen [11]. In addition, there was no statistical association between cryptosporidiosis and HIV/AIDS [11]. Recently, Certad et al. reported that Cryptosporidiosis in HIV-infected Venezuelan adults was strongly related with acute or chronic diarrhea [12]. For non – HIV infected scenarioes, Turkcapar et al studied the prevalence of Cryptosporidium infection in affected cases who are on chronic hemodialysis owing to end-period renal failure is investigated and compared with the incident rate in the healthy population [13]. According to this study, whereas 20.27% of affected cases in the dialysis group had Cryptosporidium oocysts in their stools, none of the controls had such an infection [13]. Turkcapar et al. mentioned that since hemodialysis affected cases with chronic renal failure were candidates for renal transplantation, general preventive measures against infection must be taken and these affected cases must be screened for their carrier state before transplantation [13]. In 2002, Mahdi and Ali studied the prevalence of intestinal parasitic organisms in Iraqi affected cases with sickle-cell anemia [14]. In this work, the isolation rate of Cryptosporidium species in sickle-cell affected cases (5%) was not significantly different from that in apparently healthy individuals (1.14%) [14]. In 1998, the prevalence of Cryptosporidium infection was determined in four Aymara communities in the Bolivian Altiplano, between the city of La Paz and Lake Titicaca, at an altitude of 3,800-4,200 meters [15]. In this work, sole stool specimens were randomly collected from 377 5-19-year-old students, all apparently asymptomatic and the total prevalence (31.6%) was possibly the highest reported among healthy human beings (a maximum of 9.8% and 2.0% in coprologic surveys in underdeveloped and developed countries, respectively) and one of the highest even in symptomatic cases [15]. Esteban et al. noted that such an infection prevalence was probably related to the poor sanitation conditions, contaminated water supplies, overcrowding, and close contact with domestic animals [15]. They also mentioned that continuous exposure to the parasitic organism could be related with prevention against parasitic organism-related symptoms in the pediatric population examined [15].

Concerning the environmental effect on cryptosporidiasis, the oocyst period can remain infective under cool, moist conditions for many months, especially where water temperatures in rivers, lakes, and ponds remain low but above freezing [4]. Surveys of surface water, groundwater, estuaries, and seawater pose dispelled the assumption that Cryptosporidium oocysts are present incommonly and in geographically isolated locations [4]. Numerous reports of outbreaks of cryptosporidiosis related to drinking water in North America, the UK, and Japan, where detection means are in place, indicate that water is a main vehicle for transmission of cryptosporidiosis [4].

Genetic and Molecular Biology of Cryptosporidiosis

Cryptosporiadiasis is an infection by *Cryptosporidium* spp. The most common species is *C. parvum*, an enteric pathogenic organism with a broad host spectrum including man and domestic mammals [5]. Molecular biological studies on isolates of *C. parvum* and other species pose shown that the species is likely not to be monophyletic but presents several species with different host spectra [5]. More than ten species and several genotypes pose been described so far within the genus Cryptosporidium [5]. However, the most common species is *C. parvum*, an enteric pathogenic organism with a broad host spectrum including man and domestic mammals [4]. Molecular biological studies on isolates of *C. parvum* and other species pose shown that the species is likely not to be monophyletic but presents several species with different host spectra [5]. Based on DNA marker sequences one human and various animal genotypes can be differentiated [5]. Joachim said that infections of immunocompetent affected cases with *C. parvum* were usually related with the human genotype, whereas infections of HIV-infected affected cases could also be correlated with various animal genotypes or even primarily animal pathogenic organismic species of Cryptosporidium including *C. felis*) [5].

The recent development of subtyping tools poses led to better understanding of the population genetics and transmission of Cryptosporidium in human beings [16]. The population structure of *C. parvum* and *C. hominis* is apparently more complicated than previously suggested, with the likely existence of both clonal and panmictic populations [16].

Thus, the transmission of *C. parvum* in human beings is shown to be different in different settings, with zoonotic transmission important in certain places and anthroponotic transmission in others [16]. The use of molecular tools poses also led to the detection of geographic and temporal differences in the transmission of *C. parvum* and *C. hominis*, and better appreciation of the public health importance of other Cryptosporidium species/genotypes and the frequency of infections with mixed genotypes or subtypes [16]. Xiao and Ryan said that factors involved in the transmission of human cryptosporidiosis were difficult to examine using conventional means [16]. They said that the use of molecular tools had been helpful in the assessment of the zoonotic potential of various *Cryptosporidium* spp. and sources of human infections, and had started to play a significant role in the characterization of transmission dynamic in endemic and outbreak settings [16].

Pathophysiology and Clinical Presentation

1. Basic Knowledge on the Pathogenic organism

Cryptosporidium is classified as a protozoa. The genus Cryptosporidium comprises coccidian protozoan parasitic organisms that grow and recreate within epithelial cells of the digestive organs and the respiratory tract of vertebrates. The organism was observed in the digestive glands of laboratory mice in 1907 and formally described as the species *C. muris*. Cryptosporidium species are apicomplexan parasitic organisms that infect the microvillus border of the gastrointestinal epithelium of a wide range of vertebrate hosts, including human beings [17]. Infected individuals show a wide spectrum of clinical presentations, but the pathogenic organismicity of Cryptosporidium varies with the species of parasitic organisms involved and the type, age, and immune status of the host [17]. In many animals, Cryptosporidium infections are not related with clinical signs or are related with only acute, self-limiting disease [17]. Named species of Cryptosporidium that are currently considered valid species now include *C. andersoni* (cattle), *C. baileyi* (chicken and some other birds), *C. canis* (dogs), *C. felis* (cats), *C. galli* (birds), C. hominis (human beings), *C. meleagridis* (birds and human beings), *C. molnari* (fish), *C. muris* (rodents and some other mammals), *C. parvum* (ruminants and human beings), *C. wrairi* (guinea pigs), *C. saurophilum* (lizards and snakes), and *C. serpentis* (snakes and lizards) [17]. Xiao et al said that the clarification of Cryptosporidium taxonomy was also useful for understanding the biology of *Cryptosporidium* spp., assessing the public health importance of *Cryptosporidium* spp. in animals and the environment, characterizing transmission dynamics, and tracking infection and contamination sources [17].

Cryptosporidium infects hosts including fish, snakes, birds, mice, rats, cats, dogs, squirrels, deer, horses, pigs, sheep, cattle and others [18]. Some species (e.g., rats, mice, guinea pigs) appear to pose innate resistance as their infections are asymptomatic, whereas other (e.g., ruminants) are, as are human beings, susceptible to disease [18]. Infections occur predominantly in very young (neonate) animals, only human beings seem to be susceptible at any time in their lives [18]. Although each *Cryptosporidium* spp seems host-specific there is considerable cross-infectivity [18].

Concerning the life cycle of *C. parvum*, it is monoxenous, that is, its life cycle is completed within one host [18]. The parasitic organism moves from host to host via the fecal-oral route [18]. The resistant periods created by Cryptosporidium, oocysts, are remarkably stable, and can survive for weeks to months in the environment. Mature oocysts are shed in the feces of an infected host, then through contamination of the environment, water or food, the oocysts are ingested by other suitable hosts [18]. In the gastrointestinal tract (usually the ileum or the jejunum) or the respiratory tract (which appears a more common site of infection in birds), sporozoites excyst from the oocyst and parasitize epithelial cells [18]. The sporozoites and subsequent developmental periods are seen at the lumenal epithelium of the infected tract [18]. It is now set that all life cycle periods are intracellular, surrounded by the host membrane and a thin layer of host cytoplasm [18]. However, Rosales et al. recently confirmed the existence of extracellular periods of *C. parvum* during in vitro culture on MDCK, HCT 8 and Vero cells as well as alveolar macrophages, by optic, Nomarski and transmission electron microscopy images [19]. In their work, extracellular trophozoite/gamont, periods in syzygy, zygotes and spores with eight sporozoites were seen in the supernatant of the cultures and the first ultrastructural images of extracellular periods of C. parvum were shown [19]. Rosales et al. found that the morphology of these periods, which pose characteristics similar to those of some gregarines, supported the contention that Cryptosporidium had closer affinity with gregarines [19]. They said that this study also supported the necessity of reconsidering the life cycle of Cryptosporidium and the classification within the coccidia [19].

A unique attachment organelle, occasionally called the "feeder organelle", develops at the interface between the parasitic organism cell and the host cell cytoplasm [18]. Indeed, *C. parvum* excystation and host cell invasion pose been characterized in some detail ultrastructurally, however, until recently, the biochemical and molecular basis of host-parasitic organism interactions and parasitic organism- and host-specific molecules involved in excystation, motility and host cell invasion pose been poorly understood [20]. The sporozoite differentiates into a spherical trophozoite, then asexual multiplication occurs, forming two types of meronts (or schizonts) [18]. Type I contain 6-8 nuclei, which become incorporated into 6 to 8 merozoites when the meront is mature and each merozoite is able to infect a new host cell, and then develop either into a new type I meront, or into a type II meront, which contains 4 merozoites when mature [18]. The merozoites from type II meronts also invade new host cells, but then initiate sexual multiplication by differentiating into either male (microgametocyte) or female (macrogamont) periods [18]. Upon maturation, the microgametocytes contain spermlike microgametes, which fertilize the macrogamonts [18]. The fertilized macrogamont, or zygote, then develops into an oocyst, which undergoes meiosis within the host [18]. When sporogony (meiotic sporozoite formation) is complete each oocyst contains four potentially infective sporozoites [18]. Some oocysts are shed via the feces or perhaps via respiratory secretions [18].

2. Pathophysiology of Cryptosporidiasis

The main target of *C. parvum* in the host is the intestinal epithelial cell, resulting in diarrhea, occasionally profuse and persistent, although it might also infect other organs including the gall bladder and lungs [1,5 – 7, 21]. Pathogenic organismesis involves attachment, probably via a sporozoite lectin, invasion, probably involving apical organelles, replication within a parasitophorous vacuole with the host cell membrane, causing cellular dysfunction [1,5 – 7, 21].

The enteric nervous system is a critical component of the mechanism regulating fluid secretion in the normal intestine and a key element in the pathophysiology of diarrhea [22]. Neural reflex pathways expand epithelial fluid secretion in response to *C. parvum* [22]. Moreover, the enteric nervous system poses an important role in epithelial secretion triggered by products of activated white cells during inflammation [22]. In the suckling rat model, Barbot et al .showed that *C. parvum* infection impairs net electrogenic transport across the ileal mucosa without involvement of prostaglandins, as well as trans- and paracellular permeability and leucine and glutamate absorption [23]. These results provide evidence for the development of an intestinal malabsorptive syndrome during cryptosporidiosis [23]. Barbot et al. noted that unspecific process including villous atrophy and inflammatory cytokines secretion should be regarded as possible mediators of this syndrome; however, specific mechanisms had to be considered since *C. parvum* induces a rearrangement of the host enterocyte cytoskeleton which might impaired intracellular trafficking thus reducing the membrane expression of nutrient transporters [23].

As previously said the immune status of the host is an important factor determining the susceptibility to crytosporidiasis. Those at greatest risk are immunocompromised adults and pediatric population, especially those with AIDS, pediatric population in day care, travelers to endemic regions, dairy or cattle farm workers of their families or contacts, household contacts of scenarioes or carriers, and possibly owners of infected dogs or cats or their neighbors [1, 5 – 7].

3. Clinical Presentation

The two most important species of Cryptosporidium in human beings, *C. parvum* and *C. hominis*, cause severe and chronic life-threatening gastroenteritis in immunocompromised affected cases. Clinically, most scenarioes present to the medical doctors with diarrheal disease. Owing to the recent study of Certad et al., infection was strongly related with acute and chronic diarrhea, weight loss, CD4+ counts below 100 cells/mm^3, older age in affected cases with leukopenia, and more than 5 stools per [24]. Frost et al. done a study to assess whether serological responses to Cryptosporidium antigens are related with a minimized risk of diarrhea disease in scenarioes of infection with HIV [25]. They found that acquired protective immunity to cryptosporidiasis might be important in controlling the burden of cryptosporidiasis in immunosuppressed individuals [25]. Indeed, both humoral and cellular immunity play a role in the control of this infection, but the latter plays the main role, mainly in the intestinal mucosa, however, a natural resistance to these coccidian parasitic organisms is also involved [26]. Gomez Morales and Pozio said that IgG, IgM and IgA had been detected in serum and mucosa of human beings and animals with the resolution of the infection; but also high levels of these immunoglobulins had been detected in persons with AIDS with chronic cryptosporidiasis [26]. They noted that CD4+ T-cells in HIV-positive persons were required to prevent the establishment of the infection and IFN-gamma and CD4+ T-cells could also limit the duration and the clinical presentations of the infection [26]. They also noted that it had been possible to show the important role of IFN-gamma in both the innate and acquierythrocyte mediated immunity in persons exposed to cryptosporidial infections; hence, the severity of cryptosporidiasis had been also related with the inability to create IFN-gamma [26].

The extraintestinal cryptosporidiasis among persons at advanced period of HIV infection is usually problematic because those with extraintestinal cryptosporidiasis were found to be related with poor prognosis as reported in the water-borne outbreak in Milwaukee [27]. In 1995, Lopez-Velez et al. reported that extraintestinal infection was present in 30% of the affected cases with known intestinal cryptosporidiasis [28]. Among these scenarioes, 61.5% of the affected cases with extraintestinal cryptosporidiasis had Cryptosporidium in the bile and 16.28% had it in the sputum [28]. In this report, the mean CD4+ lymphocyte count in the affected cases with extraintestinal cryptosporidiasis was 55 cells/mm^3 [28].

For immunocompetent host, the parasitic organism, which is found more commonly in pediatric population, occurs in about 2% of fecal specimens examined and seems to be closely related with generation of symptoms [29]. A serological response poses been shown [29]. In 1990, Jongsutiwes et al. reported a case of life-threatening chronic diarrhea, caused by *Cryptosporidium* spp [30]. In this case, cryptosporidiosis manifested as severe chronic diarrhea in the immunocompetent and supportive management was very important because an sucessful drug is not available at present [30].

Diagnosis of Cryptosporidiasis

Diagnosis is generally made by visualization of the oocyst form in stool by staining means, the best of which appears to be auramine and fluorescence microscopy [1, 5 – 7]. For diagnosis, a stool sample from the subject is required for staining to find the oocysts by modified Ziehl Nelson carbolfuchsin staining [1, 5 - 7].

In 1990, Anwer et al. done an interesting study to compare of saline, iodine and stained preparations in detection for cryptosporidium oocyst [31]. In this work, 300 stool samples for routine ova and parasitic organism examination were examined as saline and iodine wet preparations. The results were then compared with the Zeihl-Neelsen-modified Acid Fast staining (MAFS), as the oocysts are acid fast in character [31]. Anwer et al. found that examination with saline preparation was unable to detect any oocyst, whereas iodine preparation yielded three oocyst and stained smears with MAFS revealed five positive stool samples [31]. Microscopically, Cryptosporidium oocysts are spherical to subspherical, measuring from 4-6 mm [32]. They are occasionally referred to as "pac-man" [32]. The oocysts contain four sporozoites [32]. However, it is difficult to differentiate the species of Cryptosporidium by staining.

In addition to microscopic diagnosis, there are also other new proposed diagnostic means [33]. Serodiagnosis is an interesting alternative. Recently, Michel et al. reported a simple and economic slide agglutination test (co-agglutination test) for detecting cryptosporidial antigen in stool, serum and water [34]. The results showed that as a screening mean co-agglutination is clearly superior to enzyme-connected immunosorbent tool (ELISA) and modified Ziehl-Neelsen staining, although ELISA was more accurate [34]. Michel et al. said that the co-agglutination test was recommended for application as a new tool for detecting cryptosporidial antigen in large-scale epidemiological surveys [34]. Presently, a variety of Polymerase Chain Reaction (PCR) tools pose been described for Cryptosporidium [35]. Based on PCR technique, the species of Cryptosporidium can be classified. In 2004, Amar et al. reported the successfulness in using PCR diagnostic tool for differentiating the species of Cryptosporidium [36]. In this work, the nested-tool comprised an initial amplification using a conventional thermocycler followed by real time PCR using a LightCycler with SYBR Green I for the characterization of the amplicons [36]. This study demonstrated a novel approach to detection of Cryptosporidium species and the detection of *C. hominis* and *C. parvum* [36]. Amar et al. noted that the technique might be especially useful for the analysis of environmental samples which were likely to contain heterogeneous mixtures of *Cryptosporidium* species [36].

Pathology and Complication

C. parvum can be regarded as a minimally invasive mucosal pathogenic organism, since it invades surface epithelial cells that line the intestinal tract but does not invade deeper layers of the intestinal mucosa [37]. Nonetheless, infection can be related with diarrhea and marked mucosal inflammation [37]. In 1998, Lumadue et al. done an interesting study to characterize the histology of AIDS-related cryptosporidiosis and identify features that imply the clinical variability [38]. A retrospective analysis of HIV-positive individuals with cryptosporidiosis who underwent endoscopy was done [38]. According to this study, histologic features related with Cryptosporidium infection include a neutrophilic infiltrate in the stomach, villus blunting in the duodenum, cryptitis and epithelial apoptosis in the colon, and reactive epithelial changes in the stomach and duodenum [38]. The nature and intensity of the inflammatory response varied widely; however, duodenal biopsies from a subset of affected cases (37%) revealed marked acute inflammation that was related with concomitant cytomegalovirus infection [38]. Although duodenal infection was common (93% of individuals), infection of other sites was variable (gastric cryptosporidiosis in 40% and colonic cryptosporidiosis in 74%) [38]. Widespread infection of the intestinal tract, which included both the large and small intestine, was related with the most severe diarrheal disease [38]. Rumadue et al. said that Cryptosporidium infection created histologic evidence of gastrointestinal mucosal injury [38]. They noted that the inflammatory response to the infection was variable, and might be modified by copathogenic organisms including cytomegalovirus and the clinical presentations were influenced, in part, by the anatomic distributed apperance of the infection, with extensive infections involving both small and large intestines producing the most severe disease [38].

In spite of intensive efforts, a consistently sucessful therapy for the infection poses yet to be identified [39]. Morbidity and fatality results from ongoing loss of absorptive epithelium, which leads to villous atrophy and malabsorption and release of inflammatory mediators that stimulate electrolyte secretion and diarrhea [39].

Therapy

There is no specific therapy available, however, in the immunocompetent host the disease is self-limited, lasting from a few days to 3 weeks, and long term carriage is rare. In the immunocompromised host, infection is prolonged, occasionally asymptomatic, but might result in chronic debilitating diarrhea with dehydration, malabsorption and wasting [1, 5 – 7]. With further clarification of the mechanisms underlying enterocyte malfunction in Cryptosporidium infection, it should be possible to design rational nutritional and pharmacologic therapies to enhance nutrient and water absorption, promote the clearance of infected enterocytes, and restore normal villus architecture and mucosal barrier function [39]. As no specific efficient therapy exists, cryptosporidiosis-induced malnutrition must be taken into account when establishing a therapeutic scheme [23]. Recently, Smith and Corcoran noted that nitazoxanide was sucessful for cryptosporidiasis in immunocompetent and probably immunocompromised affected cases (with an alteration in the duration of therapy or the dosing regimen) [40]. Of set efficacy in immunocompetent affected cases, nitazoxanide is also useful for immunocompromised affected cases [40]. Zardi et al. said that in spite of a certain efficacy shown by passive immunotherapy or by some chemotherapeutic agents, including paromomycin and nitazoxanide, no significant benefit had been demonstrated [41]. An antibody therapy using bovine colostrum from cows hyperimmunised with Cryptosporidium oocysts or monoclonal antibodies against sporozoite antigens poses been developed at the researchal level mainly for persons with AIDS or with other immunodeficiencies; however, these preparations of antibodies pose shown only a limited degree of efficacy both in animals and human beings [26]. The detection of the *C. parvum* proteases involved in the host-cell interaction could lead to new therapeutic approaches using specific parasitic organism protease inhibitors in immunocompromised persons [41]. Luckily, the use of highly active antiretroviral therapy (HAART) in persons with the acquired immunodeficiency syndrome drastically minimizes the prevalence of Cryptosporidium infection [41]. This result seems to be owing to aspartyl protease inhibitors of the human immunodeficiency virus included in HAART, which directly interfere with the life cycle of the parasitic organism [41]. This favorable outcome was usually attributed to the recovery of the host immunity; however improvements from this opportunistic infection pose been demonstrated even in the absence of immunological recovery [41]. They said that the inhibitory effect of protease inhibitors on *C. parvum* growth in vitro suggested that aspartyl proteases could pose some important functions for this parasitic organism, and proteolytic activities had been demonstrated during peak periods of excystation in *C. parvum* oocysts and cysteine and serine protease classes had been functionally related with this process [41]. Smith and Corcoran said that HIV-infected affected cases on HAART had a dramatically lower incident rate of cryptosporidiasis, attributable to the effects of intestinal immune reconstitution as well as the effect on the CD4 cell count [42]. Smith and Corcoran mentioned that protease inhibitors had a direct inhibitory effect on Cryptosporidium infection, suggesting a further reason for the reduction in the incident rate of cryptosporidiasis and implying a further possible therapeutic modality [42]. In addition, Hommer et al. said that the inhibitory effect was expanded when the aminoglycoside paromomycin was combined with the protease inhibitors indinavir, ritonavir, and to a lesser extent saquinavir, compared to the protease inhibitors alone [43].

Prevention

Prevention of the cryptosporidiasis can be easily done based on the principle of basic food sanitation. The deep-rooted habit of ingestion of raw and poorly uncooked food and dirty water should be corrected. Public health measures to minimize contamination of water supplies and vigilant surveillance will minimize the risk to populations [1, 5 – 7]. Reducing behaviors favoring fecal-oral transmission, including certain sexual activities, and scrupulous hygienic practice in the day care setting would also minimize the likelihood of transmission but not eliminate it [1, 5 – 7].

References

[1] Monis PT, Thompson RC. Cryptosporidium and Giardia-zoonoses: fact or fiction? *Infect. Genet. Evol.* 2003;3:233-44.

[2] Fayer R, Morgan U, Upton SJ. Epidemiology of Cryptosporidium: transmission, detection and detection. *Int. J. Parasitol.* 2000;30:1305-22.

[3] Keusch GT, Hamer D, Joe A, Kelley M, Griffiths J, Ward H. Cryptosporidia--who is at risk? *Schweiz Med Wochenschr.* 1995;125:899-908.

[4] Fayer R. Cryptosporidium: a water-borne zoonotic parasitic organism. *Vet. Parasitol.* 2004 ;126:37-56.

[5] Joachim A. Is Cryptosporidium a zoonotic agent? *Wien Klin Wochenschr.* 2004;116 Suppl 4:2-6.

[6] Burchard GD. Clinical importance, epidemiology and laboratory diagnosis of intestinal Cryptosporidia infection. *Immun. Infekt.* 1986;14:51-7.

[7] Joachim A. Human cryptosporidiosis: an update with special empposesis on the situation in Europe. *J Vet Med B Infect Dis Vet Public Health.* 2004;51:251-9.

[8] Lima AA. Tropical diarrhoea: new developments in traveller's diarrhoea. *Curr Opin Infect Dis.* 2001;14:547-52.

[9] Wiwanitkit V. Intestinal parasitic infections in Thai HIV-infected affected cases with different immunity status. *BMC Gastroenterol.* 2001;1:3.

[10] Saksirisampant W, Eampokalap B, Rattanasrithong M, Likanonsakul S, Wiwanitkit V, Nasingkarn A, Denmasae N. A prevalence of Cryptosporidium infections among Thai HIV-infected affected cases. *J. Med. Assoc. Thai.* 2002;85 Suppl 1:S424-8.

[11] Adjei A, Lartey M, Adiku TK, Rodrigues O, Renner L, Sifah E, Mensah JD, Akanmori B, Otchere J, Bentum BK, Bosompem KM. Cryptosporidium oocysts in Ghanaian aids affected cases with diarrhoea. *East Afr. Med. J.* 2003;80:369-72.

[12] Certad G, Arenas-Pinto A, Pocaterra L, Ferrara G, Castro J, Bello A, Nunez L. Cryptosporidiosis in HIV-infected Venezuelan adults is strongly related with acute or chronic diarrhea. *Am. J. Trop. Med. Hyg.* 2005;73:54-7.

[13] Turkcapar N, Kutlay S, Nergizoglu G, Atli T, Duman N. Prevalence of Cryptosporidium infection in hemodialysis affected cases. *Nephron.* 2002;90:344-6.

[14] Intestinal parasitic organisms, including Cryptosporidium species, in Iraqi affected cases with sickle-cell anaemia. *East Mediterr Health J.* 2002;8:345-9.

[15] Esteban JG, Aguirre C, Flores A, Strauss W, Angles R, Mas-Coma S. High Cryptosporidium prevalences in healthy Aymara pediatric population from the northern Bolivian Altiplano. *Am. J. Trop. Med Hyg.* 1998;58:50-5.

[16] Xiao L, Ryan UM. Cryptosporidiosis: an update in molecular epidemiology.*Curr. Opin Infect. Dis.* 2004;17:483-90.

[17] Xiao L, Fayer R, Ryan U, Upton SJ. Cryptosporidium taxonomy: recent advances and implications for public health. *Clin. Microbiol. Rev.* 2004;17:72-97.

[18] Crytpsporidiasis. Available at *http://www.inweh.unu.edu /inweh /cryptosporidium /1x6_s2.htm*

[19] Rosales MJ, Cordon GP, Moreno MS, Sanchez CM, Mascaro C. Extracellular like-gregarine periods of Cryptosporidium parvum. *Acta Trop.* 2005;95:74-8.

[20] Smith HV, Nichols RA, Grimason AM. Cryptosporidium excystation and invasion: getting to the intestines of the matter. *Trends Parasitol.* 2005;21:133-42.

[21] Tzipori S, Ward H. Cryptosporidiosis: biology, pathogenic organismesis and disease. *Microbes Infect.* 2002;4:1047-58.

[22] Jones SL, Blikslager AT. Role of the enteric nervous system in the pathophysiology of secretory diarrhea. *J. Vet. Intern. Med.* 2002;16:222-8.

[23] Barbot L, Topouchian A, Capet C, Magne D, Huneau JF, Kapel N, Gobert JG. Cryptosporidium parvum: functional study of the intestinal malabsorption syndrome. *Ann. Pharm. Fr.* 2001;59:305-11.

[24] Certad G, Arenas-Pinto A, Pocaterra L, Ferrara G, Castro J, Bello A, Nunez L. Cryptosporidiosis in hiv-infected venezuelan adults is strongly related with acute or chronic diarrhea. *Am. J. Trop. Med. Hygienic practice.* 2005; 73:54-57.

[25] Frost FJ, Tollestrup K, Craun GF, Fairley CK, Sinclair MI, Kunde TR. Protective Immunity Related with a Strong Serological Response to a Cryptosporidium-Specific Antigen Group, in HIV-Infected Individuals. *J. Infect. Dis.* 2005; 192:618-621.

[26] Gomez Morales MA, Pozio E. Humoral and cellular immunity against Cryptosporidium infection. Current drug targets. *Immun. Endocr. Metabol. Dis.* 2002; 2:291- 301.

[27] Eisenberg JN, Lei X, Hubbard AH, Brookhart MA, Colford JM Jr. The role of disease transmission and conferred immunity in outbreaks: analysis of the 1993 Cryptosporidium outbreak in Milwaukee, Wisconsin. *Am. J. Epidemiol.* 2005; 161:62-72.

[28] Lopez-Velez R, Tarazona R, Garcia Camacho A, Gomez-Mampaso E, Guerrero A, Moreira V, Villanueva R. Intestinal and extraintestinal cryptosporidiosis in AIDS affected cases. *Europ. J. Clin. Microbiol. Infect. Dis.* 1995; 14:677-81.

[29] Casemore DP, Sands RL, Curry A. Cryptosporidium species a "new" human pathogenic organism. *J. Clin. Pathol.* 1985;38:1321-36.

[30] Jongwutiwes S, Teeravanichpong S, Kraivichian P. Cryptosporidiosis: report of a case with life-threatening diarrhea. *J. Med. Assoc. Thai.* 1990;73:234-8.

[31] Anwer F, Khan IA, Munir MA, Yousuf MO, Asghar H. Prevalence of cryptosporidium in Rawalpindi/Islamabad a comparison of saline, iodine and stained preparations. *J. Pak. Med. Assoc.* 1990;40:219-21.

[32] Cryptosporidium species. Available at *http://www2.provlab.ab.ca /bugs/webbug /parasitic organism /artifact/crypto.htm*

[33] Petry F. Laboratory diagnosis of Cryptosporidium parvum infection. *Contrib. Microbiol.* 2000;6:33-49.

[34] Michel MY, Khalifa AM, Ibrahim IR. Detection of Cryptosporidium parvum antigen by co-agglutination test and ELISA. *East Mediterr. Health J.* 2000;6:898-907.

[35] Caccio SM. New means for the diagnosis of Cryptosporidium and Giardia. *Parassitologia.* 2004;46:151-5.

[36] Amar CF, Dear PH, McLauchlin J. Detection and detection by real time PCR/RFLP analyses of Cryptosporidium species from human faeces. *Lett. Appl. Microbiol.* 2004;38:217-22.

[37] Laurent F, McCole D, Eckmann L, Kagnoff MF. Pathogenic organismesis of Cryptosporidium parvum infection. *Microbes Infect.* 1999;1:141-8.

[38] Lumadue JA, Manabe YC, Moore RD, Belitsos PC, Sears CL, Clark DP. A clinicopathologic analysis of AIDS-related cryptosporidiosis. AIDS. 1998;12:2459-66.

[39] Gookin JL, Nordone SK, Argenzio RA. Host responses to Cryptosporidium infection. *J. Vet. Intern. Med.* 2002;16:12-21.

[40] Smith HV, Corcoran GD. New drugs and therapy for cryptosporidiosis. *Curr Opin Infect Dis.* 2004; 17:557-564.

[41] Zardi EM, Picardi A, Afeltra A. Therapy of Cryptosporidiosis in Immunocompromised Hosts. *Chemotherapy.* 2005; 51:193-196.\

[42] 42. Smith HV, Corcoran GD. New drugs and therapy for cryptosporidiosis. *Curr. Opin. Infect. Dis.* 2004; 17:557-564.

[43] Hommer V, Eichholz J, Petry F. Effect of antiretroviral protease inhibitors alone, and in combination with paromomycin, on the excystation, invasion and in vitro development of Cryptosporidium parvum. *J. Antimicrob. Chemotherapy.* 2003; 52:359-564.

Chapter 11

Diseases from Marine Animal Ingestion

Anisakidosis

Anisakidosis or anisakiasis, previously known as Herring worm disease, is a disease caused by the accidental ingestion of larval nematodes (Anisakis and occasionally Pseudoterranova) in raw fish [1]. This infection is not a real tropical disease since most of the reported scenarioes are from non- tropical zones. Many temperate countries including Japan are mentioned as endemic settings for this infection. A nationwide investigation on the incident rate of anisakiasis over a period of 5 years from 1973 through to 1977 was conducted by questionaire sent to 851 main medical centers throughout Japan [2]. In that study, the number of scenarioes for all Japanese for a period of 5 years were 334 scenarioes of gastric anisakiasis and 45 intestinal anisakiasis [2]. Asaishi et al. investigated both a random group of 3,108 inhabitants of Hokkaido and 42 anisakiasis affected cases using skin test, indirect hemagglutination test, and measurement of serum IgE, demonstrating that the etiologic mechanism of acute anisakiasis involved anaphylactic reaction as well as Arthus reaction in the digestive tract [2]. Indeed, anisakiasis is still an important food-borne infectious diseases in Japan [3]. This stems from the traditional popularity among the Japanese of ingesting raw food, coupled with an increasing fondness for rare delicacies, overseas travel, and consumption of exotic food [3].

In Europe, anisakiasis is mentioned. A retrospective study on anisakiasis was carried out in France with 32 laboratories specializing in parasitology [4]. During January 1985-September 1987, 21 scenarioes of anisakiasis were diagnosed and confirmed by parasitological detection or serology, and various fish species were involved [4]. Hubert et al. said that although anisakiasis was not a main public health problem, there is a need for regulation in the fish industry and for consumer information [4]. In USA, anisakiasis is also reported. Desowitz et al. stated most infections were caused by *Phocanema* spp. and found in California and Alaska, and most were of the tissue non-invasive type [5]. They found that a characteristic symptom of the throat named "tingling throat" was manifested most scenarioes and this symptom was found to be owing to larvae of Phocanema [5]. They mentioned in that because the causative factors of child bronchial asthma in Hawaii were few and the environmental conditions were also good, asthma was surmised to be helminth-related asthma [5].

There are some recent studies on the molecular biology of anisakiasis. Anisakiasis as well as allergic and anaphylactoid reactions to *Anisakis simplex* antigens are recently identified clinical entities [6]. They are relatively common in countries with habitual raw food consumption, often in the form of large amounts of fish and sea food products [6]. According to the report of Desowitz et al., anisakis larva antigens were analyzed, a strong immunosuppressive effect was confirmed in the high molecular weight fraction (MW: greater than 10,000), whereas the existence of a substance having mutagenicity was confirmed in the low molecular weight fraction (MW: less than 10,000). Recently, the relationship between HLA class II alleles and the IgE-specific immune response to *A. simplex* allergen was studied in a defined population in Northern Spain [6]. In this work, individuals with immediate-type Anisakis hypersensitivity and healthy controls were examined for HLA-DRB1, DQB1 and DQA1 alleles by sequence-specific oligonucleotide probe typing [6]. Concerning the results, analysis of the HLA data among affected cases revealed expanded phenotypic frequencies for DRB1*1502 and DRB1*0404 compared to healthy controls and analysis of haplotypic frequencies showed that the DRB1*1502-DQB1*0601 haplotype is significantly higher in affected cases with Anisakis hypersensitivity in comparison with the control population from the same region [6]. Sanchez-Velasco et al. suggested that this haplotype could be considered to be a susceptibility factor for hypersensitivity to *A. simplex* antigens [6]. In 2001, Paggi et al .proposed combined allozyme and morphological analyses provided markers for the detection of the four sibling species of the *Pseudoterranova decipiens* complex and their nomenclatural designations [7]. In their work, new markers based on PCR-RFLP analysis were used for the detection of sibling species of the *A. simplex* complex and of another four species of the genus [7]. According to this study, genetic markers based on three diagnostic restriction enzymes permited the detection as *A. pegreffii* of a larva obtained by endoscopy in a case of human anisakidosis in Southern Italy [7]. D'Amelio et al. said that PCR-RFLP proved to be a cost-sucessful and reliable tool for the exact detection of Anisakis larvae recovered from infected human beings [8].

Concerning the life cycle, adult periods of *A. simplex* or *P. decipiens* reside in the stomach of marine mammals, where they are embedded in the mucosa, in clusters [9]. Unembryonated eggs created by adult females are passed in the feces of marine mammals [9]. The eggs become embryonated in water, and first-period larvae are formed in the eggs [9]. The larvae molt, becoming second-period larvae, and after the larvae hatch from the eggs, they become free-swimming [9]. Larvae released from the eggs are ingested by crustaceans [9]. The ingested larvae develop into third-period larvae that are infective to fish and squid [9]. The larvae migrate from the intestine to the tissues in the peritoneal cavity and grow up to 3 cm in length [9]. Upon the host's mortality, larvae migrate to the muscle tissues, and through predation, the larvae are transferred from fish to fish [9]. Fish and squid maintain third-period larvae that are infective to human beings and marine mammals [9]. When fish or squid containing third-period larvae are ingested by marine mammals, the larvae molt twice and develop into adult worms [9]. The adult females create eggs that are shed by marine mammals. Human beings become infected by ingesting raw or undercooked infected marine fish [9]. After ingestion, the anisakid larvae penetrate the gastric and intestinal mucosa, causing the symptoms of anisakiasis [9]. Recently, Klimpel et al. said that *A. simplex* was able to select definite host species depending on the locality, apparently having a very low level of host specificity [10]. They said that this could imply the wide range of different hosts that pose been recorded for this species, and could be seen as the reason for the success of this parasitic organism in reaching its marine mammal final hosts in an oceanic environment [10].

As previously described, the parasitic organism requires marine mammals for its development and the larvae are found in fishes, crustaceans and cephalopods, which are intermediate hosts. Bouree et al. noted that infestation rate was high in fishes: cod (88%), rock fish (86%), herring (88%), salmon, mackerel [1]. The risk of infection with *A. simplex* and related parasitic organisms of fish poses been recognized for some time, but it is now emerging that ingestion of material from dead parasitic organisms in food is also potentially dangerous [11]. Concerning the clinical presentations of anisakiasis, Bouree et al. studied 25 scenarioes with anisakiasis and found that most of the scenarioes complained of acute symptoms, which occurred within 12 hours of ingesting the seafood meal--epigastric pain, occlusion, diffuse abdominal pain, and appendicitis. Larvae were attached to the gastric mucosa (25 scenarioes), including an inflammatory response (erythema, oedema ulceration) [1]. In this series, diagnosis of anisakiasis is made by gastroscopy which permits removal of the worms, and cures the affected cases. In gastro-intestinal tract X-rays, edema in the mucosa, pseudo tumor formation, and filling defects (worm) were observed [1]. In chronic infections, scenarioes with intermittent feelings of ill health and abdominal pain, lasting from several weeks to months, were misdiagnosed as another intestinal disease [1]. Bouree et al noted that positive serological reactions were helpful, and surgery was needed for resection of the problematic lesion; diagnosis was made histologically by an eosinophilic granuloma, and the existence of a larva with Y shaped lateral cords [1]. Repiso Ortiga et al. studied 25 scenarioes of gastrointestinal anisakiasis and found that all the affected cases had ingested raw anchovies. Two groups were observed [11]. According to this report, the first group was composed of 10 affected cases with a gastric form of the infection, in which the main symptom was epigastralgia (90%) and oral endoscopy was done in all affected cases and the parasitic organism was detected in five (50%) [12]. The second group was composed of 15 affected cases with intestinal involvement in which the main presentations were symptoms mimicking appendicitis (80%) [12]. In this series, the most common finding of laparotomy and/or imaging tests (abdominal ultrasonography, intestinal transit, abdominal CAT) was terminal ileitis (80%) [12]. Seven affected cases underwent surgery: intestinal resection was done in four with detection of *A. simplex* in three and eosinophilic infiltration was found in all surgical specimens [12]. In this series, therapy was symptomatic in most of the affected cases and outcome was favorable in all [12]. Repiso Ortiga et al concluded that infection with Anisakis simplex should be investigated in the affected cases with abdominal pain after intake of raw fish, ileitis of unclear origin, or eosinophilic gastroenteritis [12].

In addition to digestive symptoms, allergy is another important presentation. Whereas gastric anisakiasis poses been known for several decades, the implications of *A. simplex*-related allergic disorders had not been thoroughly studied until the late 1990s [13]. Acute anisakiasis is probably caused by an inflammatory and/or allergic response in the digestive tract mucosa with abdominal pain [14 – 16]. It can also induce IgE-mediated reactions with several clinical presentations ranging from urticaria/angioedema to anaphylaxis [14 – 16]. Gastroallergic anisakiasis describes an acute hypersensitivity reaction emerging in the context of an acute parasitism by the *A. simplex* [13]. But other common allergic disorders like chronic urticaria are now being studied for a possible relationship with *A. simplex* parasitism [13]. In recent investigations, non-IgE mediated mechanisms, including the involvement of other immunoglobulin isotypes (IgG4), or non-immunological events are discussed [13]. The experience of the last several years shows that allergic hypersensitivity symptoms in gastroallergic anisakiasis are clinical events accompanying a wide range of immunologic reactions as a host response against a ubiquitous parasitic organism [13]. The resulting allergic reactions range from rapid onset and potentially lethal anaphylactic reactions to chronic, debilitating conditions [11].

For the pathology, Rosset et al. mentioned anisakiasis as a parasitic disease characterized by eosinophilic granulomas affecting the human gastrointestinal tract [14]. Infection might occur following ingestion of raw or poorly cooked fish [14]. Rosset et al. noted that affected cases generally presented with an acute abdominal syndrome mimicking a wide variety of clinical conditions, thus cringesting a diagnostic dilemma [14]. According to the report of Navarro Cantarero et al. the most common reason for seeking medical assistance was right iliac fossa pain and radiological findings of an inflammatory intestinal process were observed in 60 % of the affected cases [15]. According to this report, 75 % of the affected cases had eaten raw or insufficiently cooked fish and had eosinophilia; of these, 80 % had elevated specific IgE levels [15]. Navarro Cantarero et al. concluded that the incident rate of anisakiasis was increasing and consequently knowledge of its most characteristic clinical, radiological and laboratory presentations was important [15]. They mentioned that the most commonly affected segment of the digestive tract was the ileum and many affected cases pose symptoms of acuteabdominal pain, mimicking appendicitis or peritonitis [15]. Chronic anisakiasis results from abscesses or eosinophilic granulomas caused by parasitic organism invasion [16]. This later form can mimic appendicitis, duodenal ulcer, inflammatory bowel diseases and intestinal obstruction [16]. An early gastroduodenoscopy can confirm the diagnosis and prevent the complications [16]. However, serodiagnosis of anisakiasis is difficult since many Anisakis antigens show cross-reativity complications [16]. In childhood it is more difficult to make a right diagnosis than in the adult population [17]. Most of positive prick tests to AS correspond to pediatric population with positive prick tests to other allergens [17]. In fact many people pose high IgE titles in the absence of obvious allergic reactions to seafoods [16]. The secretor-excretory antigen shows a better specificity, recognizing the true parasitized affected cases [17]. This antigen could be used as indicator of parasitization [17].

Considering therapy for anisakiasis, Navarro Cantarero et al said that anisakiasis was a self-limiting process that usually resolves in 1-2 weeks, hence, a conservative attitude is advisable to avoid unneeded surgery [15]. Albenzadole was recently proposed as an sucessful drug for anisakiasis [18 – 19]. Recently, The activity of ivermectin and albendazole against larval Anisakis simplex was tested in vitro and in researchally infected guinea pigs [20]. Dziekonska-Rynko et al. found that the efficacy of both drugs against *A. simplex* was high in vitro and in vivo against the larvae in different organs of guinea pigs [19].

Concerning the prevention of anisakiasis, public health education should discourage the ingesting of raw fish [1]. Thorough cooking to 70 degrees Celcius or adequate freezing to -20 degrees Celcius for 72 h are the best preventive measures [1, 16]. To follow prevention rules for AS, avoid consumption of raw fish unless frozen for 48 hours or ingestion of fresh fish always cooked for more than 20 minutes at least at 60 Celcius [17]. Recently, Sanchez-Monsalvez et al. proposed a new procedure for marinating fresh anchovies and ensuring the rapid destruction of Anisakis larvae [20]. In this report, they used high food-grade acetic acid concentrations (10, 20, 30, and 40% [vol/vol] in line with the quantum satis rule) to destroy the larvae rapidly [20]. Cabrera et al. said that anisakiasis was most probable during the "El Nino" Weather Phenomenon; however, during normal conditions it was probably owing to the expand of raw fish consumption and other factors [21]. They noted that eviscerating the fish would be most adequate prevention [21]. Since anisakiasis is not an actual tropical food-borne zoonosis disease, more details are not hereby provided.

Diphyllobothriasis

Diphyllobothriasis is a tapeworm infestation. The main causative agent for diphyllobotriasis is *Diphyllobothrium latum* or fish tape worm. Similar to anisakiasis, this disease is not an actual tropical disease. In 1998, Nozaki et al. done a brief survey of common intestinal parasitic organisms in the Tokyo Metropolitan Setting [22]. They found an apparent expand in the incident rate of infections with the tapeworms *D. latum* and proposed that this might just be a implyion of affected cases gathering at a few facilities for therapy [22]. Muratov et al. reported that results of epidemiological studies of diphyllobothriasis in the Lower part of the Amur watershed had demonstrated that the disease nosogeographic range covered the entire region [23]. They noted the potential risk of invasion of human beings and animals by the tapeworms exists all over the aforementioned setting [23]. They found that the season of invasion coincided with the period of migration of calico and humpback salmon which were additional hosts of Diphyllobothriidae [23]. They concluded that invasion occurred outside the Amur freshwater setting; thus the real disease foci are absent in the Lower part of the Amur watershed and said that this was owing to the fact that the disease was not induced by wide fish tapeworm, but by a marine or estuarine-marine species [23].

However, there is a recent report of diphyllobothriasis in India [24], implying the importance of travelling medicine. *D. latum* is endemic to Scandinavia, western Russia, and the Baltics, though it is now also present in North America, especially the Pacific Northwest [25]. In additional to *D. latum*, there pose been twelve other species of this genus reported to infect human beings, especially *D. dendriticum* (the salmon tapeworm), which poses a much larger range (the whole northern hemisphere) [25].

The principal species causing Diphyllobothriasis is *D. latum*, known as the broad or fishy tapeworm, or broad chess tapeworm [25]. *D. latum* is the longest tapeworm in human beings, averaging ten meters long [25]. Adults can shed up to a million eggs a day. *D. latum* is a pseudophyllid cestode that infects fish and mammals [25]. It is morphologically very similar to other members of the genus Diphyllobothrium, but can occasionally be distinguished by host [25]. Morphologically, adult Diphyllobothrium worms range from 1-12 meters in length, pose proglottids that are wider than their length, and discharge ovoid eggs that measure 60 mm X 40 mm [26]. Considering the life cycle of *D. latum*, the life cycle begins with an infected host discharging eggs into a freshwater environment that contains susceptible crustaceans and fish [26]. After the eggs hatch, the embryonic flatworms are ingested by water fleas; in these crustaceans, the first larval period develops [26]. When a fish devours the infected crustacean, a second larval period develops, and this larva is infective to the definitive hosts [26]. The juvenile worm develops to maturity in the small intestine of the definitive host and, within 3-5 weeks, begins to create eggs [26]. Adult diphyllobothrium worms might survive longer than 10 years [26]. Another interesting infection relating to diphyllobothriasis is sparganosis. By definition, sparganosis is an infection of animals, including fish and man, with a developmental period of Diphyllobothrium [27]. This period poses recently been referred to as a plerocercoid but the name sparganum poses persisted [27]. Hence, infection of fish or other animals with the plerocercoid larvae is sparganosis. Fish-ingesting mammals, including man, are the final hosts [27]. In addition to ingesting the marine fish, ingesting frog or snake meat and using frog or snake meat as a poultice are other commons sources of sparganosis.

The clinical symptoms of diphyllobothriais are varied. For acute infestation, the digestive symptoms are predominant. In 2001, Terramocci et al described six scenarioes which were diagnosed within a period of 4 months, which all originated from the setting of Lake Como (Lombardy region) in italy [28]. In this report, all cases had previously eaten raw perch fillets [28]. Four individuals complained of gastrointestinal signs and symptoms, whereas two were asymptomatic [28]. In 1989, et al. reported 7 scenarioes of diphyllobothriasis in Korea [29]. According to this report, all of the affected cases had the history of ingesting several kinds of raw marine fishes, and they had never been abroad [29]. In addition, one of the scenarioes experienced abdominal pain and 6 experienced natural discharge of a chain of worm segments, but none revealed any sign of anemia [29]. For chronic infestation, anemia is an important presentation. Megaloblastic anemia owing to *D. latum* is well documented in hematology [30 – 31]. This type, tapeworm anemia, is one of the two well-known infection-related anemia, hookworm anemia and tapeworm anemia. For the scenarioes with megaloblastic anemia, the blood picture can show megalocyte and hypersegmented neutrophil [32].

Considering sparganosis, the clinical presentation is usually the mass at different site of body. As a nature of accidental infection, the central nervous system involvement in sparganosis is reported. According to the recent report of Wiwanitkit considering 34 scenarioes of sparganosis, the infections were ocular (17 scenarioes), subcutaneous (ten scenarioes), central nervous system (five scenarioes), auricular (one case), pulmonary (one case), intraosseous (one case) and intraperitoneal (one case) [33]. Of these 34 scenarioes, 14 had risk behaviour reported, 12 had a history of drinking impure water, five had a history of ingesting frog or snake meat and two had a history of using frog or snake meat as a poultice [33]. Some scenarioes had more than one risk factor [33]. Wiwanitkit concluded that most scenarioes of sparganosis in Thailand presented with superficial ocular mass problematic lesions and the main risk behaviour in Thailand is drinking water contaminated with the infective organism [33]. Wiwanitkit noted that some scenarioes of serious deep visceral sparganosis had also been reported [33]. It can be seen that although sparganosis exists in tropical countries including Thailand it is not related to marine fish consumption.

For diagnosis of diphyllobothriasis [34], stool examination for the parasitic organism's egg is a useful tool. In addition, infected individuals occasionally pass visible segments of worm (proglottids) in stool and can be a clue for diagnosis. In additional, complete blood count might reveal anemia with large red blood cells, which can be a supportive evidence for diagnosis of chronic diphyllobothriasis [32]. Problems with the specific detection of these parasitic organisms from the fish hosts prompted the development of a series of nucleic acid probes [35]. Use of the polymerase chain reaction proved to be quick, accurate and requires little skill, once developed [35].

For therapy, niclosamide or praziquantel are given in a sole dose to treat the tapeworm infection [33]. Albendazole is another sucessful drug. Studies of the effects of the anthelminthic agent albendazole on the tissues of *D. latum* in vivo showed large shapeless protrusions of the outer tegumental cytoplasm on the surface of strobila, the mitochondrial degeneration in the tegumental cells and their nucleolar material segregation [36]. After in vitro therapy cavitary formations in the outer tegumental syncytium, muscular fascicle loosening, decreased glycogen levels, and altered secret granules in the vitellaria were found [36]. Vitamin B-12 injections or supplements might be required for the therapy of megaloblastic anemia. For sparganosis, surgical removal is the best therapy [33].

For prevention, food sanitation is still the key point. To complete its development from egg to adult worm the parasitic organism poses to pass through two obligatory intermediate hosts before invading its final host [37]. At each period critical ecological parameters pose to be encountered, among them oxygen concentration, light intensity and temperature [37]. The first intermediate host, which remained unknown for a long time, is one of many copepod species; the second hosts are fish, notably species belonging to the genera Esox. Perca and Lota [37]. Hence, control of disease should focus on each step in the life cycle. Survey of contamination in the intermediate host is an sucessful mean for disease control. Health education should also be accompanied with getting rid of the infection. Since diphyllobothriasis is not an actual tropical food-borne zoonosis disease, more details are not hereby provided.

Other Seafood Zoonosis

Many species of parasitic organisms from marine organisms are known to be zoonotic. Marine zoonotic infections in human beings result from consumption of contaminated edible tissues or products of seafood or, to a lesser extent, from physical contact with contaminated seafood [38 – 40]. Worldwide, over 50 species of helminth parasitic organisms from fishes, crabs, crayfishes, snails, and bivalves are known to create human infections [38 – 40]. This is closely related with the tradition of ingesting raw fishes and invertebrates [38]. In addition to the two described worms, attention to worldwide pollution of the coastal marine environment poses focused primarily on toxic algal blooms and pathogenic organismic bacteria that multiply in nutrient-rich waters [39]. However, massive but unseen amounts of feces from human beings, their pets, and their domesticated animals are discharged, dumped, or carried in runoff, bringing encysted zoonotic protozoan parasitic organisms to estuaries and coastal waters [39]. They can contaminate bathing beaches, are filtered and concentrated by shellfish eaten by human beings and marine mammals, and infect a wide range of marine animal hosts, resulting in morbidity and fatality to some populations [39]. Giardia, Cryptosporidium and Toxoplasma are the three well-described protozoa for this problem [39]. Some viruses are also documented as important marine food zoonosis. Shellfish and oysters are the two foods with high contamination [41]. Apart from the hepatitis A virus (HAV) the Norovirus (NLV) is becoming more significant [41].

Recent trends in mariculture include technical improvement in seed generation and importation of large quantities of various species of culture seedlings [38]. Drastic expand in the supply of seedlings of selected fish species poses resulted in changes in culture means and created parasitic organism problems on a much larger scale [38]. Most helminth zoonoses are rare and invoke only slight to moderate injury; however, some are more prevalent and pose serious potential health hazards [40]. Worldwide, the mainity of seafood zoonoses occur along coastal regions where seafood products are commonly consumed [40]. An efficient quarantine system to prevent and control introduction and spread of marine parasitic organisms urgently needs to be set [38]. Continuing improvements in transportation, technology, and food handling, however, permit fresh seafood to be shipped throughout the world; thus, the potential for acquisition of parasitic infections from marine products is not limited to coastal populations [40]. Although the number of documented scenarioes continue to expand, the overall risk of human infection is slight [40]. Deardorff said that the increasing exploitation of the marine environment by human beings, changing dietary habits incorporating natural seafood dishes, including sushi and sashimi), and trend to minimize cooking times when preparing seafood products, all increasd the chances of becoming infected with the pathogenic organismic organisms [40].

References

[1] Bouree P, Paugam A, Petithory JC. Anisakidosis: report of 25 scenarioes and review of the terature. *Comp. Immunol. Microbiol. Infect. Dis.* 1995;18:75-84.

[2] Asaishi K, Nishino C, Totsuka M, Hayasaka H, Suzuki T. Studies on the etiologic mechanism of anisakiasis. --2. Epidemiologic study of inhabitants and questionaire survey in Japan. *Gastroenterol. Jpn.* 1980;15:128-34.

[3] Kamiya M, Ooi HK. Current status of food-borne parasitic zoonoses in Japan. *Southeast Asian J. Trop. Med. Public Health.* 1991;22 Suppl:48-53.

[4] Hubert B, Bacou J, Belveze H. Epidemiology of human anisakiasis: incident rate and sources in France. *Am. J. Trop. Med. Hyg.* 1989;40:301-3.

[5] Desowitz RS. Human and researchal anisakiasis in the United States. Hokkaido Igaku Zasshi. 1986;61:358-71.

[6] Sanchez-Velasco P, Mendizabal L, Anton EM, Ocejo-Vinyals G, Jerez J, Leyva-Cobian F. Association of hypersensitivity to the nematode Anisakis simplex with HLA class II DRB1*1502-DQB1*0601 haplotype. *Hum. Immunol.* 2000;61:314-9.

[7] Paggi L, Mattiucci S, D'Amelio S. Allozyme and PCR-RFLP markers in anisakid nematodes, aethiological agents of human anisakidosis. *Parassitologia.* 2001 ;43 Suppl 1:21-7.

[8] D'Amelio S, Mathiopoulos KD, Brandonisio O, Lucarelli G, Doronzo F, Paggi L. Diagnosis of a case of gastric anisakidosis by PCR-based restriction fragment length polymorphism analysis. *Parassitologia.* 1999;41:591-3.

[9] Anisakiasis. Available at *http://www.dpd.cdc.gov/dpdx/HTML/Anisakiasis.htm*

[10] Klimpel S, Palm HW, Ruckert S, Piatkowski U. The life cycle of Anisakis simplex in the Norwegian Deep (northern North Sea). *Parasitol. Res.* 2004 ;94:1-9.

[11] Audicana MT, Ansotegui IJ, de Corres LF, Kennedy MW. Anisakis simplex: dangerous--dead and alive? *Trends Parasitol.* 2002;18:20-5.

[12] Repiso Ortega A, Alcantara Torres M, Gonzalez de Frutos C, de Artaza Varasa T, Rodriguez Merlo R, Valle Munoz J, Martinez Potenciano JL. Gastrointestinal anisakiasis. Study of a series of 25 affected cases. *Gastroenterol. Hepatol.* 2003;26:341-6.

[13] Daschner A, Pascual CY. Anisakis simplex: sensitization and clinical allergy. *Curr. Opin. Allergy Clin. Immunol.* 2005;5:281-5.

[14] Rosset JS, McClatchey KD, Higashi GI, Knisely AS. Anisakis larval type I in fresh salmon. *Am. J. Clin. Pathol.* 1982;78:54-7.

[15] Navarro Cantarero E, Carro Alonso B, Castillo Lario C, Fernandez Gomez JA. Diagnosis of Anisakis infestation: experience in our environment. *Allergol. Immunopathol .(Madr).* 2005;33:27-30.

[16] Gani F, Lombardi C, Senna G, Mezzelani P. Anisakiasis: a borderline disorder. *Recenti. Prog. Med.* 2001;92:302-6.

[17] Valls A, Pascual CY, Martin Esteban M. Anisakis and anisakiosis. *Allergol. Immunopathol.* (Madr). 2003;31:348-55.

[18] Moore DA, Girdwood RW, Chiodini PL. Therapy of anisakiasis with albendazole. *Lancet.* 2002;360:54.

[19] Dziekonska-Rynko J, Rokicki J, Jablonowski Z. Effects of ivermectin and albendazole against Anisakis simplex in vitro and in guinea pigs. *J. Parasitol.* 2002;88:395-8.

[20] Sanchez-Monsalvez I, de Armas-Serra C, Martinez J, Dorado M, Sanchez A, Rodriguez-Caabeiro F. A new procedure for marinating fresh anchovies and ensuring the rapid destruction of Anisakis larvae. *J. Food Prot.* 2005 ;68:1066-72.

[21] Cabrera R, Del Pilar M, Altamirano T. Anisakidosis a marine parasitic zoonosis: unknown or emerging in Peru? *Rev. Gastroenterol. Peru.* 2004;24:335-42.

[22] Nozaki T, Nagakura K, Fusegawa H, Ando Y. Brief survey of common intestinal parasitic organisms in the Tokyo Metropolitan Setting. Kansenshogaku Zasshi. 1998;72:865-9.

[23] Muratov IV, Posokhov PS. Epidemiologic characteristics of diphyllobothriasis in the lower Amur River valley. *Med. Parazitol* (Mosk). 1989;:53-7.

[24] Pancharatnam S, Jacob E, Kang G. Human diphyllobothriasis: first report from India. *Trans. R. Soc. Trop. Med. Hyg.* 1998;92:179-80.

[25] Diphyllobothriasis. Available at en.wikipedia.org/wiki/Diphyllobothriasis

[26] Connectlater D. Diphyllobothriasis. Available at *http://www.emedicine. com /med /topic571.htm*

[27] Sparganosis. Available at *http://www.5mcc.com/Assets/SUMMARY/TP0861.html*

[28] Terramocci R, Pagani L, Brunati P, Gatti S, Bernuzzi AM, Scaglia M. Reappearance of human diphyllobothriasis in a limited setting of Lake Como, Italy. *Infection.* 2001 Mar-Apr;29(2):93-5.

[29] Lee SH, Chai JY, Hong ST, Sohn WM, Huh S, Cheong EH, Kang SB. Seven scenarioes of Diphyllobothrium latum infection. *Kisaengchunghak Chapchi.* 1989 ;27:213-6.

[30] Anaemia and the fish-tapeworm. *Lancet.* 1977 ;1:292

[31] Pathogenic organismesis of the tapeworm anaemia. *Br. Med. J.* 1976;2:1028.

[32] Wiwanitkit V. Abnormality in clinical hematologic test for infectious diseases. *Lampang. Hosp. Bull.* 2004; 25: 148-162.

[33] Wiwanitkit V. A review of human sparganosis in Thailand. *Int. J. Infect. Dis.* 2005 Jul 13;

[34] Yamane Y. Laboratory diagnosis of protozoan and parasitic infections. 2. Helminthiasis. b. Diphyllobothrium infections. Rinsho Byori. 1998 *Nov;Suppl.* 108:215-9.

[35] Dick TA, Dixon BR, Choudhury A. Diphyllobothrium, Anisakis and other fish-borne parasitic zoonoses. *Southeast Asian J. Trop. Med. Public Health.* 1991;22 Suppl:150-2.

[36] Molodozhnikova NM, Volodin AV, Bakulina NG. The action of albendazole on the broad tapeworm. *Med. Parazitol.* (Mosk). 1991;(6):46-50.

[37] von Bonsdorff B, Bylund G. The ecology of Diphyllobothrium latum. Ecol Dis. 1982;1:21-6.

[38] Ogawa K. Marine parasitology with special reference to Japanese fisheries and mariculture. *Vet. Parasitol.* 1996;64:95-105.

[39] Fayer R, Dubey JP, Lindsay DS. Zoonotic protozoa: from land to sea. *Trends Parasitol.* 2004 ;20:531-6.

[40] Deardorff TL. Epidemiology of marine fish-borne parasitic zoonoses. *Southeast Asian J. Trop. Med. Public Health.* 1991;22 Suppl:146-9.

[41] Schrader C, Reetz J, Suss J. Food-borne human pathogenic organismic viruses and their molecular detection with special concern of noroviruses and hepatitis A virus in mussels. Berl Munch Tierarztl Wochenschr. 2003;116:496-505.

Chapter 12

Botulism

Introduction to Botulism

Botulism is a group of infections disease caused by a bacterium namely *Clostridium botulinum*. The two main forms of this infection are food-borne and wound botulism [1]. Food-borne botulism is an important food-borne infectious disease with high fatality [2]. Food-borne botulism is reported in many developing countries [3 - 4]. Food-born botulism is a fatal bacterial infection. The contamination of causative bacterium in home-canned food is the most common cause of outbreak [5]. The causative agent, *C. botulinum*, is a rod bacterium producing subterminal endospore. This pathogenic organism grows best in low oxygen conditions. However, the knowledge on the climatic preference of this germ is limited. To diagnosis of infected scenarioes, detection of botulinum toxin in blood or body fluid samples is the gold standard [6]. For therapy, specific antitoxin is recommended [7].

Geographical Approach for Botulism

Geographical pathology for botulism is of interest. Wiwanitkit recently reported the geological geographical parameters of this pathogenic organism in Thailand [8].

The objective of this study was to determine ecology of *C. botulinum* from previous reported outbreaks [8]. According to this work, the averages (mean +/- SD) for % soil moisture, % humus and pH were 0.6 +/- 0.1% (range 0.5-0.7), 3.0 +/- 0.2% (range 3-3.2) and 5.2 +/- 0.1 (range 5.1-5.4), respectively [8]. All outbreak settings shared the same sandy loam soil type. It can imply that provinces with this type of ecology might pose sites harboring *C. botulinum* [8]. However, there is no report on the contamination of the organism and its relation to atmospheric geography in Thailand. Here, the author done this retrospective study in order to document the atmospheric geographical parameters of the organism in Thailand based on the data of the previous outbreaks. This study is designed as a retrospective study. A literature review of the papers concerning botulism in Thailand was done, using the database of published works cited in the Index Medicus and Science Citation Index. The author also reviewed the published works in all 256 local Thai journals, which are not included in the international citation index. The key word for finding is "Botulism". The geographical setting of each outbreak was recorded and used for further analysis for the geographical parameters the geographical parameters of each setting including average temperature, average rainfall and average humidity are determined according the basic reference geography documents [9]. Description statistical analysis was done where it was proper. There are 4 reports on the outbreaks of food-bone botulism in Thailand [10 – 13]. The geographical setting and parameters are presented in Table 1. Concerning the geographical parameters, the average (mean ± SD) for average temperature, average rainfall and average humidity are 30.0 $\pm$ 1.6 Degree C (range 28 – 32), 1125.0 $\pm$ 95.7 mm (range 1,000 – 1,200), 75.0 $\pm$ 4.1 % (range 70 – 80), respectively.

It can be shown that there are a specific range of geographical parameters for the organism. This might be the optimal condition for this pathogenic organism. According to this study, it can imply that any provinces with this pattern of geographical parameters might be silent sites harboring of *C. botulinum*. The provinces within the range of the described climatic parameters are those in the eastern and western part of the Northern Region and those in the Western Region (Table 2). However, some limitations of this study should be noted. The actual comparative survey for the soil contaminant in different provinces should be done. Since the proposed hypothesis might change the present knowledge on this pathogenic organism further studies to verify are required. Occurring of disease also depends on other factors including the ingesting habits of local populations especially ingesting the canned preserved food). The generalization of the results must be carefully considered.

Table 1. Geographical setting and parameters of food-bone botulism outbreak in Thailand

Reference	Setting	Parameters		
		Average temperature (Degree C)	Average rainfall (mm)	Average humidity (%)
[10]	Nan	30	1200	75
[11]	Tak	32	1000	70
[12]	Lampang	28	1100	80
[13]	Nan	30	1200	75
Mean		30	1125	75
Standard deviation		1.6	95.7	4.1
range		28 – 32	1,000 – 1,200	70 – 80

Table 2. Geographical climatic parameters in different provinces in Thailand

Parameters	Example of provinces
Average temperature (Degree C)	
24	Phuket, Trang, Rayong
26	Loei, Chiangmai, Suratthani, Phuket
28	Lampang, Chiangrai, Maehongsorn
30	Nan, Phrae, Uttaradit
32	Tak, Uthaithani
34	Kanchanaburi, Petchaburi, Srakaew
Average rainfall (mm)	
900	Roiet, Srisaket, Maposesarakham, Buriram
1000	Tak, Tak, Uthaithani
1100	Lampang, Lamphun, Maehongsorn
1200	Nan, Phrae, Uttaradit
1300	Suratthani, Phuket, Phanga
1400	Trad, Ranong
Average humidity (%)	
65	Roiet, Srisaket, Kalasin, Khonkaen
70	Tak, Kanchanaburi, Uthaithani
75	Nan, Phrae, Uttaradit
80	Lampang, Lamphun
85	Trad, Ranong, Pattalung

Social Geographical Parameters in Previous Outbreak of in Thailand

1.Introduction

Botulism is a group of infectious disease caused by a bacterium namely *Clostridium botulinum* [14]. The two main forms of this infection are food-borne and wound botulism Food-borne botulism is an important food-borne infectious disease with high fatality [15]. Food-borne botulism is reported in many developing countries [3 - 4]. In Thailand, outbreaks of food-borne botulism pose been documented for years. The causative bacterium is a contaminant in roots and shoots of many plants.

Social epidemiology is a subject in which it poses a strong interest. Here, descriptive social geography of previous outbreaks in Thailand is summarized and presented. In addition, the most interesting aspects of botulism, which relate to the technology, economics and regulation of the food chain and to consumer behavior, are also captured. Details on how outbreak occurs and how they are dealt with are also presented.

Here, the author done a mini-study in order to document the social geographical parameters of the organism in Thailand based on the data of the previous outbreaks. This study is designed as a retrospective study. A literature review of the papers concerning botulism in Thailand was done, using the database of published works cited in the Index Medicus and Science Citation Index. The author also reviewed the published works in all 256 local Thai journals, which are not included in the international citation index. The key word for finding is "Botulism".The geographical setting of each outbreak was recorded and used for further analysis for the geographical parameters of each setting including average income, gross provincial product and HDI are determined according the basic reference geography documents. Description statistical analysis was done where it was proper. As previously mentioned, there are 4 reports on the outbreaks of food-bone botulism in Thailand [10 – 13]. The geographical setting and parameters are presented in Table 3. Concerning the geographical parameters, the average (mean ± SD) for average income, gross provincial product and HDI are 42,037.0 + 7,162.7 baht/year (range 31,500 – 47,529), 24,217.0 + 10,180.4baht/year (range 15,907 - 36,692) and 0.66 + 0.04 (range 0.63 – 0.72), respectively.

Food-born botulism is a fatal bacterial infection. The contamination of causative bacterium in home-canned food is the most common cause of outbreak [16]. The causative agent, *C. botulinum*, is a rod bacterium producing subterminal endospore. This pathogenic organism grows best in low oxygen conditions.

According to the described in the early section, the optimal climatic factors for the germ is defined. However, the main question left is how the social geography pattern for the organism in Thailand is.

Here, the author summarizes the social geographical parameter for this organism in Thailand. According to this study, a specific range of social geographical parameters for the organism can be derived. For disease prediction purpose, the detected parameters might be the optimal condition for this pathogenic organism. According to this study, it can imply that any provinces with this pattern of geographical parameters might be silent sites harboring of *C. botulinum*.

Table 3. Geographical setting and parameters of food-bone botulism outbreak in Thailand

Reference	Setting	Parameters		
		Average income (baht)1,2	Gross provincial product (x 106baht /year)2	Quality of life index (HDI)2
Wongwatcharapaiboon	Nan3	44,559	15,907	0.63
Chotechuang	Tak3		28,362	0.72
Swaddiwudhipong	Lampang3	31,500	36,692	0.67
Bhosiri	Nan3	47,529		0.63
			15,907	
		44,559		

[1] US Dollar equal to 40 baht

[2] Data from of Thailand National Economics and Social Development Bureau (www.nesdb.go.th)

[3] located in the eastern and western part of the Northern Region of Thailand

The provinces within the range of the described geological parameters are those in the eastern and western part of the Northern Region and those in the Eastern Region of Thailand. These findings are concordant with the conclusion from climatic geography study in the previous section of this chapter.

At this point, there is a left question to be answered and that is why there poses never been any outbreak in the Eastern Region of Thailand. The answer might be the cultural or spiritual context difference. The provinces in the eastern and western part of the Northern Region belong to the Lanna Thai subculture; however the provinces in Eastern Region do not. One of cultural differences is the ingesting behavior difference. In the Northern Region, there is a tradition of food preservation by canning. Whereas the practice in the Eastern region is ingesting fresh bamboo shoot. This can be the clue for the absence of outbreaks of botulism in some provinces although the climatic and social geography parameters of those settings are prone for outbreak.

2. How Did Outbreak Occur?

2.1. Local Technology: Risk for Outbreak?

In Thailand, agriculture is still the main occupation. Thai people can derive to vegetables through several channels. The local well-known motto, "Nai Nam Mee Pla Nai Na Mee Khao" or "There are fishes in the water and there are rice in the paddy field" can imply the abundance of foods in Thailand. A large number of indigenous vegetables exist in tropical rain forests along jungle tracks, roadside or in wild weeds [17]. The local Thai people living in these settings are usually aware of these vegetables and use them as components in their daily dishes. Home gardens provide a supplementary source of essential nutrients in the family diet through products obtained from self-sustainable farming of vegetables grown in pots and school gardens [17]. The group activities of "Farm Housewife" include the preservation of vegetable as, fermented, pickled, dehydrated or dried, and occasionally canned products [17]. These processes also play a role in local vegetable supply [17].

Canned foods in local Thai communities are similar to those in other developing countries. The main problem as bacterial contamination can be expected.

In 1987, Imwidthaya et al. [18] proposed for the high microbial contamination in some common fresh and preserved foods in Bangkok and mentioned for the requirements of quality control in food generation. Indeed, the home canned-food is the main causes of the food-borne botulism in the literature [19]. Renewed educational efforts combined with a comprehensive food control plan would significantly improve the control of botulism in high-risk populations [20].

At present, Thai FAO poses strict control for food manufacturers and this can minimize the problem of food contamination. Although there are many control means for food no danger in Thailand, problems owing to home-preserved food can be seen. Considering the four outbreaks in Thailand, all outbreaks including the most recent outbreak, are owing to home-canned food without quality control process. Home-canned bamboo shoot is a well-known local wisdom for the people in the northern region of Thailand. One of the problems of the local wisdom in food preservation is lack for the standard and quality control. Hence, the educational plan for the local population is needed. The good example is the plan set by the local college in Uttaradit province in northern region of Thailand [21]. However, the outbreak in the distance setting is still occurreing.

Home canned bamboo shoot is a local technology that can help the local population to derive sufficient food in dry season. Contamination in the canned food owing to the lack of good machinery can be expected. Owing to the local geography in some settings of Thailand especially for provinces in Northern region, the growth of possible contaminated bacteria can be promoted. The practice without good standard can be the great risk. If the knowledge on good manufacturing practice is introduced to local villagers, home canned bamboo shoot will become a not dangerous and valuable local wisdom of Thailand.

2.2. Biological Aspect Contributing to Outbreak

As previously described, the causative agent of botulism is a soil-contaminant bacterium which can be destroyed by heat [22]. Good cleaning of bamboo shoot and boiling before canning can help get rid of contamination. However, if these processes are not done, the contamination will be left. In the can, lacking of air, the bacteria will be full grow, giving off the problematic toxin-botulinum, causing food-borne botulism. This toxin cannot be gotten rid of by simple boiling or hingesting [23]. Hence, although the consumer boils or heats contaminated canned bamboo shoot, they are at risk for getting the toxin and Botulinum disease can then result.

2.3 Economical Aspect Contributing to Outbreak

The impact of economics on outbreak of botulism is noted. The relation between low economical status and expanded risk for some food-borne infectious diseases including botulism, Salmonella, and *Escherichia coli* is proposed [24]. The possible explanation is that limitation of income leads the people to preserve the food for the longest consumption possible. However, the purpose of home canned food preparation in Thailand is not totally related to the economical reason. Basically, the local practice for food preservation in Thailand is usually drying in air, which requires no specific machine, owing to the nature of tropical countries. The preservation by canning is occasionally hard to practice by local population. Of interest, the settings where the outbreaks occurred are not the provinces with low average income. In addition, these provinces are classified in a group of provinces with high gross provincial product.

2.4. Regulation of the Food Chain: is there any Problem Leading to Outbreak?

Regulation of the food chain, especially for processing, is important in control of food-borne botulism. Thailand poses long enforced laws and regulations on food no danger. The responsibility for food control is shared between different agencies and ministries under the following laws and regulations [25]. Ministry of Public Health, Ministry of Agriculture and Cooperatives, Ministry of Industry and Ministry of Commerce are the main authorities in Thailand involving in regulation of food. Food Act B.E. 2522 (1979) and Controlling Importation and Exportation Goods Act. B.E. 2522 (1979) are the two important Acts covering the food manufacturing process in Thailand [25]. Surveillance of food no danger in food industrial brings good quality of Thai food product and the food products from Thailand are accepted from many countries around the world.

Hence, what is the problem in the case of botulism outbreak in Thailand? As previously mentioned, all of the outbreaks were owing to home-canning, which is not covered by the present Acts. Basically, public health Acts, in any countries, do not strictly cover the daily ingesting habit. There is no regulation on how to eat for the people since it is the human rights to eat. The regulations on community level for controlling of local food generation in village are possible but it is impossible to regulate on the home level. The best prevention choice should be health education as previously described.

2.5 Consumer Behavior: Which Contribute to Outbreak?

As previously mentioned, cultural or spiritual context might lead the occurrence of outbreak in provinces in the eastern and western part of the Northern Region of Thailand. A tradition of food preservation by canning, which is different from other regions might be the clue. Concerning the local products in the list of the project namely OTOP or "one tambon one product" (www.thaitambon.com), supported by Thai Government, the canned bamboo shoot can be proved as the local wisdom of northern Thai people and can be a rooted consumer behavior [26]. Hence, it is not surprising as to why the previous outbreaks confined in the northern region occurred, but not in other regions where there are similar climatic and social geographical parameters.

3. How Were the Outbreaks Dealt With?

3.1. Medical and Public Health Response

Since there is a system of disease surveillance in Thailand, many infectious diseases including botulism are in the list of the diseases under surveillance to be reported. Once the outbreak occurred, the affected cases were delivered to the local hospital and got the diagnosis. Usually, the presumptive diagnosis of botulism was based on clinical history and physical examination [10 – 13]. Transferring to the tertiary hospital for proper management was done in each outbreak [10 – 13]. Final diagnosis was done according to the results reported by the reference medical laboratory. The record and announcement of botulism as well as disease control was the next step. For disease control process, the practical protocols in medical epidemiology were usually followed. Detection of the source of outbreak, control of pathogenic organism, tringesting of affected cases as well as prevention for further transmission were done [27].

3.2. Social Response to the Outbreak

Usually, the news of outbreaks are repeated broadcast via several media including radio and television in the acute pposese of outbreak. The avoidance of bamboo shoot ingesting by general population as a panic response to the news can be observed. Indeed, this pattern of response is a classical pattern of psychological response to any outbreak [28 – 29]. Many health education plans are broadcast to the local population at this pposese. However, the continuous of this event is not observed and the social response when the time pass is usually decrease.

Concerning political dimension, some clear directions in responding to the outbreak in medicine: 1) strong refind and education campaigns; 2) close contact with political colleagues, interest groups and the community; 3) a national strategy which enjoins diverse interest groups, with courage, rationality and compassion are also used [30]. Public information campaigns on television and launching of several funding for refind on botulism in Thailand are the good examples of those political responses to the most recent outbreak.

4. Social Geography of the Last Recent Botulism Outbreak in Thailand

4.1. Description of the Outbreak

On 19 March 2006, two scenarioes of food-borne botulism were reported to the Center of Disease Control of Thailand (Thai CDC), Thai Ministry of Public Health.The affected cases are a group of 143 local populations of Ban Laung District, Nan Province who had an appointment for ingesting food together at a Buddhist temple festival. All affected cases had nausea, vomiting after ingesting canned bamboo shoots and developed respiratory and neurological symptoms. The affected cases were sent to the community hospital and referred to the tertiary hospitals in Nan province and Bangkok. The affected cases received symptomatic therapy, antitoxin, which was provided from USA, and were discharged from the hospital within 4 weeks. There are totally 2 mortality scenarioes. Investigation of the outbreak was undertaken by the Local Food Authorities (LFA) and the Public Health Officer (PHO), assisted by epidemiologists from the Thai CDC. To try to find the source of the infection, food histories were collected and the premises inspected. The source of this outbreak is confirmed as the canned bamboo shoots.

4.2.Social Risk Factors for the Recent Botulism Outbreak in Thailand

The source of infection in this outbreak is similar to other previous reports in Thailand and other countries. Home canned food is the main cause of food-borne botulism in many developing countries [3 – 4]. As previously described, ingesting of canned bamboo shoots is a rooted traditional ingesting in Northern Thailand. Of interest, a tradition of ingesting together at a local temple festival can be seen in this outbreak. This is another interesting consumption habit in the Southeast Asia [31]. If there is no sanitation control, this tradition can be a risk for common source type food-borne outbreak [32].

Generally, the food brought to the temple is usually a considered good food by the local population. In this outbreak, the problem is not the bacterial but toxin contamination. The botulinum toxin is a heat stable toxin in nature and cannot be successfully got rid of by a simple local cooking mean. Hence, the problem of local food generation, not the cooking practice, is the main cause of this outbreak.

As previously said, the local food generation is occasionally not covered by the Food Act B.E. 2522 (1979). Since there is a booming of local food generation owing to the OTOP policy [26], more strict control on the local food generation process in Thailand is required.

5. Social Impacts of Recent Botulism Outbreak in Thailand

Even though this outbreak was very limited in a place, there was an extensive coverage in the media. There are a heap of external pressures on local authorities under pressure from the mass media to make quick decisions on the problem. In Thailand, the radio channels, television channels and local press angled their stories in a way that heightened concern about botulism and source of pathogenic organism. As a result of the scare of bolulism spreading in the community and the recent response of the Thai society to this outbreak is a widespread panic on bamboo shoot ingesting. In the first week after the outbreak is broadcast on the public media, the general population refused to eat bamboo shoot and this directly affected the bamboo shoot business. The bamboo shoot sellers noted their income was minimized to 90% [33]. It takes for months, even with the health education from Thai Ministry of Public Health for Thai people to return to ingesting bamboo shoots. However, there is no specific additional local food control Acts corresponding to this outbreak. Nevertheless, this outbreak brings health concerns of Thai people on dangerous food-borne diseases, which are common in Thailand. The financial consequences of this outbreak, quality control for local food generation and health promotion, can be expected [33]. Also, this outbreak brings new experience to Thai medical society and world medical society in coping with botulism, which can be a bioterrorism.

6. Recommendations

For disease control measures, the substantial coverage in the local media, and lack of knowledge on how to handle the situation from the local authorities, led to the implementation of initial control measures, some of which were not very rational and without much purpose. Basic health knowledge on problematic tropical disease should be provided to the local health care workers who are faced with the real diseases. Efforts should be made to disseminate this information to officials and beneficiaries.

Provision of sanitary facilities for local food creaters could decrease the potential risk for pathogenic organism contamination of their food. Surveillance and control of disease poses to be supported by laws that make implementation of control measures possible. In this particular outbreak, botulism was not considered a main public health risk, however, similar preparedness plans should be improved to deal with more contagious and threatening food borne diseases.

Clinical Presentation of Botulism

Botulism is a rare paralytic disease caused by a neurotoxin created from the spore-forming bacterium *C. botulinum* and in rare scenarioes *C. butyricum* and C. baratii [34]. Almost all human scenarioes of botulism are caused by one of three serotypes (A, B, or E) [35]. Botulism poses 4 naturally occurring syndromes: food-borne, wound, infant botulism, and adult intestinal toxemia [34] However, the author hereby focus on food borne botulism. As previously mentioned, botulism is a food borne neurotoxin based disease. The blockage of the neurological system is the hallmark of botutism. Respiratory muscle paralysis is the important finding and becomes the leading cause of mortality for botulism [36].

Ouagari et al. reported an epidemiologic and descriptive study of 11 affected cases suffering from botulism, admitted at the Infectious Diseases department and in the Medical Intensive Care Unit of Ibn Rochd University Hospital, from August, the 10th to October, the 1st, 1999 [37]. According to this outbreak, clinical diagnosis of botulism was made, at the admission, on ocular signs (diplopia, ptosis), swpermiting troubles and/or muscle weakness but there was no fever, no trouble of conscience and normal reflexes [37]. However, most of the other reports indicated the severe respiratory and cardiovascular collapse as clinical presentations [10 - 13, 38 - 39]. Internal and external ophthalmoplegia, bilateral facial nerve palsies, and descending muscle weakness culminating in a sudden respiratory arrest is common [40]. The history of ingestion of home canned food is the clue for clinical diagnosis for all scenarioes.

Diagnosis and Therapy of Botulism

Food borne botulism is a relatively rare clinical syndrome, whose symptomatology is generally highly distinctive [41]. The medical doctors of various specialties should be familiar with the symptoms of botulism because its symptoms concern the nervous system, the organ of sight and the gastrointestinal system [41]. Laboratory proof of botulism is set with the detection of toxin in the affected case's serum, stool, or wound [35]. A strain of Clostridium botulinum can be isolated from feces which, after culture, by the dialysis mean. Indeed, an enzyme-connected immunosorbent tool (ELISA) for Clostridium botulinum type A and type B toxins is proposed for diagnostic accuracy in scenarioes of infant botulism [42]. However, it seems to be useless in the case of severe sudden food-borne botulism. As previously mentioned, the good history of ingesting home canned food is the main clue for diagnosis. Electrophysiologic testing can be especially helpful when biotool studies are negative [35]. The most consistent electrophysiologic abnormality is a small evoked muscle action potential in response to a sole supramaximal nerve stimulus in a clinically affected muscle [35]. Posttetanic facilitation can be found in some affected muscles [35].

Supportive therapy by intermittent mechanical ventilation and specific trivalent antitoxin administration are recommended for food-borne botulism scenarioes. Basically, botulinum neurotoxins are the most toxic proteins for human beings and are classified as category A toxins. Sucessful antitoxin is required for therapy. If the therapy is promptly given, the prognosis is usually good [38 – 39]. However, in the setting with lack for specific antitoxic, the high fatality can be expected [10 – 13]. It should also be noted that the polyvalent antiserum normally contains A, B and E antitoxins, hence, the F toxin might still be failed for therapy [43]. As an evidence, Richardson reported on a case of type F botulism in southern California.and concluded that administration of bivalent botulinum antitoxin did not halt progression of paralysis [44]

Prevention for Botulism

Insufficient cooking time and temperatures, storage in heat-shrinked plastic wrap, and inadequate refrigeration likely contributes to *C. botulinum* spore survival, germination, and toxin generation [45]. Hence, food sanitation and good canned food generation system are the two core for prevention of this disease. Similar to other food borne disease, surveillance for food contamination is required. In spite of adequate understanding of how foodborne botulism might be avoided, outbreaks still occur, specifically among people consuming certain high-risk or ethnic foods [46].

Botulism vaccine is the hope for prevention of botulism. In the early 1930s, a formalin-inactivated toxoid against botulinum neurotoxin was first tested in human beings [47]. In 1965, a pentavalent botulinum toxoid (PBT) received Investigational New Drug (IND) status under the Centers for Disease Control's IND 161 (for at-risk workers), and in 1991 under the United States Army's Office of the Surgeon General IND 3723 (for military deployment) [47]. In 2008, Balwin et al. reported the first E. coli-derived vaccine that sucessfully neutralizes each of the seven botulinum neurotoxins serotypes [48]. Pier et al said that a recombinant containing a double amino acid substitution, R363A Y365F (termed BoNT/A(RYM) represented a viable vaccine candidate for a holotoxoid against botulism [49]. However, the aim for developing of vaccine for vaccine is expected for the terrorism more than the prevention of food borne botulism.

References

[1] Horowitz BZ. Botulinum toxin. *Crit. Care Clin.* 2005;21:825-39.

[2] Bohnel H, Gessler F. Botulinum toxins--cause of botulism and systemic diseases? *Vet. Res. Commun.* 2005 Might;29(4):313-45.

[3] Obana M. Food-borne botulism. Ryoikibetsu Shokogun Shirizu. 1999;(23 Pt 1):456-9.

[4] Robinson RF, Nahata MC. Management of botulism. *Ann.. Pharmacother.* 2003 Jan;37(1):127-31.

[5] Todd EC. Epidemiology of foodborne diseases: a worldwide review. *World Health Stat Q.* 1997;50(1-2):30-50

[6] Delbos V, Abgueguen P, Fanello S, Brenet O, Alquier P, Granry JC, Pichard E. Botulism, a clinical diagnosis. *Presse Med.* 2005 Mar 26;34(6):449-54.

[7] Jones RG, Corbel MJ, Sesardic D. A review of WHO International Standards for botulinum antitoxins. *Biologicals.* 2006 Sep;34(3):223-6.

[8] Wiwanitkit V. Ecology of Clostridium botulinum causing food-borne botulism in Thailand. *Southeast Asian J. Trop. Med. Public Health.* 2006 Nov;37(6):1160-2.
[9] Senanarong S, Ngamnisai N. Thai Atlas. Bangkok: Aksorncharroenthus, 1986
[10] Vongvatcharapaiboon P, Sriprasert P, Nanthawas S, Wisessuk T, Leksiriwilai S, Thanawong A. Report on disease surveillance on food borne botulism from local canned bamboo roots in Ban, 2541 B.E. *Thai Month Dis. Sur.*1999; 30(6): 169-178.
[11] Swaddiwudhipong W, Wongwatcharapaiboon P. Foodborne botulism outbreaks following consumption of home-canned bamboo shoots in Northern *Thailand. J. Med. Assoc. Thai.* 2000; 83: 1021-1025
[12] Chotechuang Y, Puavilai T, Worawongprapa P. Silent murder related with home-canned-preserved bamboo shoots. *Lampang Hosp. Bull* .2005 Jan-Jun; 26(1): 90-104
[13] Bhosiri P. Thai FDA warns "danger of canned bamboo roots". *Thai FDA News* 20 March 2006.
[14] Horowitz BZ. Botulinum toxin. *Crit. Care Clin.* 2005;21:825-39
[15] Bohnel H, Gessler F. Botulinum toxins--cause of botulism and systemic diseases? *Vet. Res. Commun.* 2005;29:313-45.
[16] Todd EC. Epidemiology of foodborne diseases: a worldwide review. *World Health Stat Q.* 1997;50:30-50
[17] FAO. Vegetables and food security. Available at *http://www.fao.org/docrep /004/ ac145e/AC145E06.htm* Access on August 4, 2006
[18] Imwidthaya S, Komolpis P, Anukarahanonta T, Chaiprasert A. Microbial contamination in some common fresh and preserved foods in Bangkok. *J. Med. Assoc. Thai.* 1987;70:463-7.
[19] Pinilla J, Gimeno C, Gomez A, Anton F, Labarga P, Campos C, Gil A, Milazzo A. Clinico-epidemiological study of botulism poisoning in La Rioja (1979-1990). *Enferm. Infecc. Microbiol. Clin.* 1993;11:202-5.
[20] Hauschild AH, Gauvreau L. Food-borne botulism in Canada, 1971-84. *CMAJ.* 1985;133:1141-6.
[21] Clinic Technology Uttaradit Rajabhat University. Bamboo shoot canning. Available at clinictech.uru.ac.th/acnainn1.htm Access on August 4, 2006
[22] Obana M. Food-borne botulism. Ryoikibetsu Shokogun Shirizu. 1999;(23 Pt 1):456-9
[23] Schantz EJ, Sugiyama H. Toxic proteins created by Clostridium botulinum. *J. Agric. Food Chem.* 1974;22:26-30.
[24] Roberts JA. Economic aspects of food-borne outbreaks and their control. *Br. Med. Bull.* 2000;56(1):133-41.
[25] Thai FAO. Strengthening Official Food No danger Control Services. Presented at Second FAO/WHO global forum of food no danger regulators Bangkok, Thailand, 12-14 October 2004
[26] ThaiTambon. Available at *www.thaitambon.com/tambon/tprodtsrc.asp* Access on August 4, 2006
[27] Health Prevention Agency Centre for Infections. Communicable disease and health prevention quarterly review: January to March 2005: from the Health Prevention Agency Centre for Infections. *J Public Health* (Oxf). 2005;27:303-7

[28] Boulougouris JC, Rabavilas AD, Stefanis CN, Vaidakis N, Tabouratzis DG. Outbreak faintness: a psychophysiological investigation. *Psychiatr. Clin.* (Basel). 1981;14(4):215-25

[29] Maunder R, Hunter J, Vincent L, Bennett J, Peladeau N, Leszcz M, Sadavoy J, Verhaeghe LM, Steinberg R, Mazzulli T. The immediate psychological and occupational impact of the 2003 SARS outbreak in a teaching hospital. *CMAJ.* 2003;168:1245-51

[30] Blewett N. Political dimensions of AIDS. AIDS. 1988;2 Suppl. 1:S235-8

[31] Buddha-Dhamma Meditation Center. Buddhist Festival. Available online at *www.buddhistbmc.org/forum* Access on September 16, 2006

[32] Thorn CJ. Bacterial food-borne zoonoses. *Rev. Sci. Tech.* 2000;19:226-39.

[33] Thai Ministry of Public Health. Botulism Webboard. Available online at *http://wwwnno.moph.go.th/botulism* Access on September 16, 2006

[34] Bielec D, Modrzewska R. Botulism in the past and today--clinical aspects. Przegl *Epidemiol.* 2007;61(3):505-12.

[35] Cherington M. Clinical spectrum of botulism. *Muscle Nerve.* 1998 Jun;21(6):701-10.

[36] Bielec D, Modrzewska R. Botulism in the past and today--etiological, epidemiological and pathogenic organismic aspects. *Przegl Epidemiol.* 2007;61(3):513-8.

[37] Ouagari Z, Chakib A, Sodqi M, Marih L, Marhoum Filali K, Benslama A, Idrissi L, Moutawakkil S, Himmich H. Botulism in Casablanca. (11 scenarioes). *Bull. Soc. Pathol. Exot.* 2002 Nov;95(4):272-5.

[38] Horwitz MA, Marr JS, Merson MH, Dowell VR, Ellis JM. A continuing common-source outbreak of botulism in a family. *Lancet.* 1975 Nov 1;2(7940):861-3.

[39] Zanon P, Pattis P, Pittscheider W, Roscia G, De Giorgi G, Sacco G, Vötter K, Stockner I, De Giorgi F, Wiedermann CJ. Two scenarioes of foodborne botulism with home-preserved asparagus. Anasthesiol Intensivmed Notfallmed Schmerzther. 2006 Mar;41(3):156-9.

[40] Paterson DL, King MA, Boyle RS, Pond SM, Whitby M, Wright M, Henderson A. Severe botulism after ingesting home-preserved asparagus. *Med. J. Aust.* 1992 Aug 17;157(4):269-70.

[41] Chwaluk P, Chwaluk A. Diagnostic difficulties in foodborne botulism--case reports and literature review. *Przegl Lek.* 2007;64(4-5):348-51.

[42] Dezfulian M, Hatheway CL, Yolken RH, Bartlett JG. Enzyme-connected immunosorbent tool for detection of Clostridium botulinum type A and type B toxins in stool samples of infants with botulism. *J. Clin. Microbiol.* 1984 Sep;20(3):379-83.

[43] Fernández RA, Ciccarelli AS, Arenas GN, Giménez DF. First outbreak of botulism caused by Clostridium botulinum subtype *Af. Rev. Argent. Microbiol.* 1986;18(1):29-31.

[44] Richardson WH, Frei SS, Williams SR. A case of type F botulism in southern California. *J. Toxicol. Clin. Toxicol.* 2004;42(4):383-7.

[45] Villar RG, Shapiro RL, Busto S, Riva-Posse C, Verdejo G, Farace MI, Rosetti F, San Juan JA, Julia CM, Becher J, Maslanka SE, Swerdlow DL. Outbreak of type A botulism and development of a botulism surveillance and antitoxin release system in Argentina. *JAMA.* 1999 Apr 14;281(14):1334-8, 1340.

[46] Slater PE, Addiss DG, Cohen A, Leventhal A, Cposessis G, Zehavi H, Bashari A, Costin C. Foodborne botulism: an international outbreak. *Int. J. Epidemiol.* 1989 Sep;18(3):693-6.

[47] Smith LA, Rusnak JM. Botulinum neurotoxin vaccines: past, present, and future. *Crit. Rev. Immunol.* 2007;27(4):303-18.

[48] Baldwin MR, Tepp WH, Przedpelski A, Pier CL, Bradshaw M, Johnson EA, Barbieri JT. Subunit vaccine against the seven serotypes of botulism. *Infect. Immun.* 2008 Mar;76(3):1314-8.

[49] Pier CL, Tepp WH, Bradshaw M, Johnson EA, Barbieri JT, Baldwin MR. Recombinant holotoxoid vaccine against botulism. *Infect. Immun.* 2008 Jan;76(1):437-42.

Chapter 13

Brucellosis and Milk No Danger

Introduction to Botulism

Brucellosis is an important bacterial infection. It can be classified as an important food borne infectious disease. Franco et al. said that human brucellosis still presented scientists and clinicians with several challenges, including the understanding of pathogenic organismic mechanisms of *Brucella spp*, the detection of markers for disease severity, progression, and therapy response, and the development of improved therapy regimens [1]. Microbiologically, Brucellae are tiny, aerobic, slow growing, catalase and oxidase positive Gram negative coccobacilli or small rods, which might reach man through exposure to tissues of mammalian hosts via cuts or aerosols, or as food infections mostly through dairy products [2]. Brucellae can very long-lasting infections in all mammalian social animals, including ungulates, canids, and rodents [2].

Guerra said that Brucellae were likely to be among the toughest organisms to control through public health and agricultural policies, even involving detection-slaughter strategies [2].

Brucellosis poses a worldwide distributed apperance that mainly affects persons working with domestic animals and animal products [3]. In spite of being controlled in many developed countries, the disease remains endemic in many parts of the world, including Latin America, the Middle East, Spain, parts of Africa, and western Asia [3]. Basically, the disease is transmitted to human beings through the ingestion of raw milk or non-pasteurized cheese contaminated with one of the four Brucella species pathogenic organismic to human beings [3]. In Australia with its crucial beef export component, several priority settings can be identified including the completion of the Brucellosis and Tuberculosis Eradication Campaign [4].

Brucellosis is considered a public health problem of meat and milk. Brucellosis is an important milk borne infectious disease [5]. Another important milk borne infectious disease is tuberculosis. At present, tuberculosis and brucellosis pose been controlled, but milk-borne outbreaks of salmonellosis and campylobacter enteritis owing to raw or defectively pasteurised milk are common and might be increasing in number [6]. Trends in the epidemiology of human brucellosis in Germany was studied by Dahouk et al [7]. According

to this work, the epidemiology of brucellosis in Germany poses evolved from an endemic occupational disease among the German population into a travel-related foodborne zoonosis, primarily affecting Turkish immigrants [7]. Dahouk et al. said that prolonged diagnostic delays and high case fatality called for targeted public health measures for brucellosis [7]. Minas studied the epidemiology of brucellosis in Central Greece and found that the incident rate of human brucellosis in the setting was 32.49 scenarioes/100,000 inhabitants [8]. According to this work, males, owing to their professions, were affected more often by brucellosis than females and the mainity of the scenarioes were attributed to direct contact with animals or their products [8]. In 2006, Lee et al. studied on seroprevalence of brucellosis among risk population in Gyeongsangbuk-do, Korea and indicated in higher seroprevalence rate among veterinarians than among livestock workers and artificial inseminators [9]. Because veterinarians might be exposed to this high risk, Lee et al. proposed that sucessful working guidelines for veterinarians to guard against brucellosis must be developed [9]. Meky et al. studied epidemiology and risk factors of brucellosis in Alexandria governorate, Egypt [10]. Meky
et al. found that working with animals, breeding goats, and ingesting ice cream bought from street vendors were significantly related with brucellosis [10]. Based on these epidemiological studies, brucellosis is still a focused infectious threat. In this article, the author will focus the presentation on brucellosis and milk no danger.

Clinical Presentation of Brucellosis

Brucellosis is a zoonotic disease that is related with chronic serious sequelae in human beings. Exposure to aborted home-owned animals and consumption of home-made milk products obtained from bazaars or neighbors are identified as probable sources of human brucellosis infections [11]. Brucellosis affected cases usually present with histories of fever, chills, night swingesting, weakness, malaise and headache [12]. However, those symptoms are usually not specific. Sit et al. studied history and clinical presentation of brucellosis in Turkish scenarioes. According to this work, transmission route was the consumption of unpasteurized fresh cheese, and unboiled milk. The most common symptoms were recorded as chills, fever, and arthralgia (81%). Splenomegaly and hepatomegaly were the predominant physical examination signs [13]. Lulu et al. studied clinical pattern of 400 scenarioes of brucellosis in Kuwait and found that the main features on presentation, irrespective of the history of the disease, were fever, swingesting, headache, rigors, arthralgia, myalgia, and low back pain whereas hepatosplenomegaly was present in 41 % [14]. In addition, the haematologic findings were not specific and hepatic dysfunction was common [14]. Vogt et al. studied another case series of 9 affected affected cases in Lausanne [15]. Vogt et al. said that the time from first symptoms to diagnosis varied between 10 days and 5 months in spite of classical initial symptomatology (fever, rigors, weakness) [15]. This delay probably implies why 6 of 9 affected cases were admitted because of septic complications: meningitis, arthritis, orchi-epididymitis, and endocarditis [15].

Of several complicated brucellosis, neurobrucellosis is widely mentioned.

Lubani et al. reported nine pediatric population with neurobrucellosis [16]. The clinical presentation included meningitis in six affected cases, one with encephalitis, one with meningoencephalitis and one with meningomyeloencephalitis [16]. Haji-Abdolbagi et al. studied another case series of 31 neurobrucellosis scenarioes [17]. Haji-Abdolbagi et al. found that meningitis and meningoencephalitis were the most common form of neurobrucellosis [17]. Haji-Abdolbagi et al. concluded that the differential diagnosis of neurobrucellosis was wide, however, the disease should be ruled out in all affected cases who develop unimplyed neurological symptoms, especially in those who live in endemic settings [17]. Koussa et al. reported another case series [18]. In this series, initial clinical presentations consisted of meningoencephalitis, acute and subacute meningitis, intracranial hypertension, polyradiculoneuritis with albumin-cell dissociation, and transverse myelitis and lumbar epidural abscess with root involvement [18]. Kochar studied another case series and reported that the clinical profile of neurobrucellosis could mimick to commonly seen neurological infective diseases like tubercular meningitis, viral encephalitis, aseptic meningitis, cerebral malaria and viral encephalopathy [19]. They also note that serum and cerebrospinal fluid testing for brucella antibody titer was an important test for the diagnosis [19].

Arthritis is another interesting rare presentation of brucellosis. The clinical features of acute Brucella arthritis were reported in a prospective study of 58 Iraqi affected cases [20]. According to this work, polyarthritis occurred in 33, was migratory in ten, additive in 23 and symmetrical in ten [20]. Brucellar arthritis in 12 pediatric population were also studied by Gómez-Reino et al. [21]. Fever and oligoarthritis of the lower extremities were the most common clinical findings [21]. Another case series were also studied by Benjamin et al. [22]. A subacute presentation with peripheral oligoarthritis predominantly affecting hips or knees was common in this case series [22]. Blood and joint fluid culture can be useful for diagnosis. Finally Sankaran-Kutty et al. concluded that the commonest site was the sacroiliac joint, and brucellosis had to be differentiated from tuberculosis as an important cause of backache [23].

Considering orchi-epididymitis, brucella infection should be considered in the differential diagnosis of affected cases presenting with epididymo-orchitis from an endemic setting [24]. It is not rare to find brucella organisms in urine during acute infection. However, it commonly presents with orchi-epididymitis, and, rarely, with granulomas in the urinary tract [25]. For brucellosis induced orchi-epididymitis, almost all affected cases pose fever, swelling, and scrotal pain, but urinary symptoms can be seen in a few scenarioes [26]. Memish and Venkatesh studied case series of brucellar epididymo-orchitis in Saudi Arabia and reported that all affected cases complained of swollen painful testicles whereas other presenting symptoms included undulant fever, chills, arthralgia, dysuria and haematuria [27]. Memish and Venkatesh said that careful history, a meticulous physical examination and a rapid laboratory evaluation help in diagnosis. Memish and Venkatesh also stated that leucocytosis was not an atypical feature of brucellar epididymo-orchitis, and, hence, could not be used for differentiating it from the nonspecific variety [27]. Of interest, relapse can be seen. In proper therapy is the main cause of relapse [28].

Concerning endocarditis, it carries a high fatality rate if undiagnosed or misdiagnosed [29]. Brucella endocarditis is a destructive process of the aortic valve with abscess formation that commonly leads to heart failure [30]. The development of a new valvar problematic lesion and bulky vegetations seen on echocardiography can help identify Brucella endocarditis occurring during systemic brucellosis [31]. Brucella endocarditis, although a rare complication of brucellosis, is the main cause of mortality related to this disease [32]. Fatality of Brucella endocarditis poses been decreased significantly by a medical-surgical approach to therapy [30].

Diagnosis and Therapy of Brucellosis

Diagnosis of brucellosis can be done by microbiological test. The history of travel to endemic countries along with exposure to animals and exotic foods are usually critical to making the clinical diagnosis [33]. Various other febrile diseasees, e.g. malaria, tuberculosis, typhoid fever and tularemia might present with the same symptoms [34]. Basically, diagnosis is usually based on indirect serological tests including serum agglutination test, complement fixation or the Coombs test [34]. The serum agglutination test can be used for a first screening and complement fixation or Coombs' test will confirm its results, however, these 'conventional' serological tests lack sensitivity and specificity [34 - 35]. A definite diagnosis requires the isolation of Brucellae from blood, bone marrow or other tissues. *B. melitensis*, *B. abortus*, *B. suis* and *B. canis* are the four main isolates [35]. Mantur et al. said that laboratory testing is indispensable for diagnosis, hence alertness of clinician and close collaboration with microbiologist were essential even in endemic settings to correctly diagnose and treat this protean human infection [33]. Enzyme-connected immunosorbent tools can be used for screening and confirmation of brucellosis, however, molecular diagnosis is the most useful tool for confirmation [34]. Various tools pose been developed and evaluated for use in human and animal brucellosis [36]. PCR-ELISA and real-time PCR tools are good examples [36]. Differential PCR-based tools tend to be more complex and consequently more difficult to perform [37]. Several strategies pose been explored to differentiate among Brucella species and strains, including locus specific multiplexing, PCR-RFLP, arbitrary-primed PCR, and ERIC-PCR [37]. The disease might be overlooked and misdiagnosed because of the difficult diagnosis and the absence and lack of experience with laboratory testing [38].

Considering therapy for brucellosis, combined antibiotic regimen as doxycycline-rifampicin or doxycycline-streptomycin is recommended. Skalsky et al. reported that there were significant differences in sucessfulness between currently recommended therapy regimens for brucellosis [39]. Sakran et al. suggested that the standard therapy for acute and chronic brucellosis was a combination of doxycycline with a second drug including rifampicin or gentamicin, in order to cure, prevent complications and relapse [40]. Skalsky et al. done a metanalysis and found that overall failure was significantly higher with doxycycline-rifampicin compared to doxycycline-streptomycin, mainly owing to a higher rate of relapse [39]. Skalsky et al suggested that the proper therapy should be with dual or triple regimens including an aminoglycoside [39]. Pappas et al. suggested that only the combination of doxycycline with gentamicin could be considered therapeutically adequate and cost sucessful and this concern was a main obstacle in the utilization of quinolones for brucellosis [41]. At present, some new antibiotics are also trialed for therapy for brucellosis. There are evidences that meropenem and azithromycin implementation can result in more rapid and full normalization of the bactericidial and energy systems of the researchal animals peripheral blood cells [42]. For new hope, new means of delivery including gentamicin-loaded microparticles, neutralisation of the environment where Brucella resides and use of novel antibiotics including trigecycline might be future choices [43].

Prevention for Brucellosis

Environmental, social, economic and behavioral factors prevent the eradication of brucellosis from many countries [44]. As a food borne disease, proper and comprehensive control of foodstuffs, above all of milk and milk products is required [44]. Vaccine against brucellosis is a proposed preventive mean [45]. Historically, the first sucessful Brucella vaccine was based on live *B. abortus* strain 19, a laboratory-derived strain attenuated by an unknown process during subculture [46]. This induces reasonable prevention against *B. abortus*, but at the expense of persistent serological responses [46]. A continuous development of brucellosis poses been occurring for years. In 1986, an orally administrable brucellosis vaccine, Brucella suis strain 2 vaccine was developed in China and was sucessful in animals [47]. Olsen and Stoffregen reported that although vaccination was probably the most economic control measure, administration of currently available vaccines alone was not sufficient for elimination of brucellosis in any host species [48]. Olsen and Stoffregen mentioned that development of not dangerousr and more efficacious vaccines alone, or combined with enhancements or expanded empposesis on other regulatory plan components, could pose tremendous impact on reducing the worldwide prevalence of brucellosis and the related zoonotic infections [48]. Nicolette said that whereas vaccination of human beings might be useful in control of brucellosis in some high-risk occupations, the ultimate success was dependent upon reduction of this zoonosis in natural hosts and this was most sucessfully accomplished by widespread use of vaccination [45].

Milk No Danger

Since milk is an important beverage that is drunk worldwide. The milk no danger becomes a global public health concern. Dairy biotechnology is fast gaining ground in the setting of altering milk composition for processing and/or animal and human health by employing nutritional and genetic approaches [49]. Modification of the primary structure of casein, alteration in the lipid profile, expanded protein recovery, milk containing nutraceuticals, and replacement for infant formula offer several advantages in the setting of processing [49]. The contamination of milk is another focus at present. Several chemicals and microbes can be determined as important contaminants in milk [50].

The dairy farm environment and animals on the farm serve as important reservoirs of pathogenic organismic and commensal bacteria that could potentially gain access to milk in the bulk tank via several pathways [51]. Pathogenic organismic gram-negative bacteria can gain access to bulk tank milk from infected mammary glands, contaminated udders and milking machines, and/or from the dairy farm environment [51]. This can be the cause of many milk borne infectious diseases. Oliver et al. noted that the control of microbial quality of bulk tank milk was required because (1) outbreaks of disease in human beings had been traced to the consumption of unpasteurized milk and pose also been traced back to pasteurized milk, (2) unpasteurized milk was consumed directly by dairy creaters, farm employees, and their families, neighbors, and raw milk advocates and by a large segment of the population via consumption of several types of cheeses manufactured from unpasteurized milk, (3) entry of food-borne pathogenic organisms via contaminated raw milk into dairy food processing plants could lead to persistence of these pathogenic organisms in biofilms, and subsequent contamination of processed milk products and exposure of consumers to pathogenic organismic bacteria, and (4) pasteurization might not completely destroy all foodborne pathogenic organisms in milk and inadequate or faulty pasteurization would also not destroy all foodborne pathogenic organisms [52]. Hence, the routine monitoring of bacteria obtained from bulk tank milk might be an important tool for detecting farm-level trends in antimicrobial resistance on dairy farms [53]. For evidence, Jayarao and Wang studied the prevalence of gram-negative bacteria in bulk tank milk [54]. According to this work, organisms including Agrobacterium radiobacter, Bordetella spp., Comamonas testosteroni, Listonella damsela, Ochrobactrum anthropi, and Oligella urethralis were isolated from bulk tank milk [54]. Berge et al noted that bulk milk *Escherichia coli* and Salmonella could be valuable to monitor the dynamics of antimicrobial resistance in dairy milk generation [53]. Jayarao et al. reported that an expand in the frequency of isolation of *Staphylococcus aureus* and *Streptococcus agalactiae* was significantly related with an expanded bulk tank somatic cell count [55]. Jayarao et al. mentioned that there was low correlation between different bacterial counts and bulk tank milk with low (<5000 cfu/mL) standard plate count also had a significantly low level of mean bulk tank somatic cell count (<200,000 cells/mL), preliminary incubation count (<10,000 cfu/mL), laboratory pasteurization count (<100 cfu/mL), coagulase-negative staphylococci and environmental streptococcal counts (<500 cfu/mL), and noncoliform count (<200 cfu/mL). Coliform count was less likely to be related with somatic cell or other bacterial counts [55]. Jayarao and Henning stated the requirement for educational plans for dairy creaters to be informed about the risks related with consumption of raw milk [56]. In addition to on – farm surveillance, additional voluntary oversight of farm practices, including monitoring of and controlled access to raw milk supplies on the farm could further contribute to public food no danger [57]. If dairy creaters in all scenarioes had voluntary plans in place to adequate inventory, monitoring, and control access to raw milk supplies, the outbreaks probably can pose been prevented [57].

Important Non Brucellosis Milk Borne Diseases

1. Milk Borne Tuberculosis

Tuberculosis is a very well – known infection in medicine. Bovine tuberculosis poses never mentioned as an important milk borne tuberculosis in the past [58]. Basically, before pasteurization was widely used, milk was the principal foodstuff by means of which tuberculosis was passed from cattle to human beings-indeed it could be said that it was the only sucessful vector that carried the bovine bacterium to the human organism [59]. Intestineiérrez García said that the case of milk borne infectious disease had a more serious impact with graver consequences than did meat borne disease [59]. de la Rua-Domenech mentioned that most scenarioes of zoonotic tuberculosis diagnosed in the UK were attributed to reactivation of long-standing latent infections acquired before widespread adoption of milk pasteurization [60]. de la Rua-Domenech also noted that continuing on-farm consumption of unpasteurized cows' milk and retail sales by approved establishments of unpasteurized milk and dairy products were the two significant risk of *Mycobacterium bovis* infection [60].

2. Milk Borne Q Fever

Q fever is an important zoonosis [61]. Q fever is caused by the gram-negative bacterium Coxiella burnetii, occurs worldwide, and affects both human beings and animals [62]. Ruminants are considered to be the main source of infection of human beings, with the main route of infection being through inhalation of the organism of fine-particle aerosols [62]. Q fever is also classified as a milk borne zoonosis [63]. Consumption of raw goat milk and its products are the main risks for Q fever [64]. Epidemiological studies pose been interpreted as C. burnetii being a significant pathogenic organism causing clinical disease through ingestion of milk [65]. In 2005, Kim et al. reported that more than 94% of samples of bulk tank milk from U.S. dairy herds tested were contaminated [66]. Milk pasteurization is an important control mean for this disease [61]. Stringency of milk pasteurization poses been set on requirements for *C. burnetii* as being the most heat-resistant organisms of public heath importance [65].

C. burnetii resides and replicates in the host s monocytes and macrophages [67]. The developmental cycle of *C. burnetii* includes macrocellular and microcellular forms and the formation of spore-like bodies [67]. Infection in human beings is often asymptomatic, but an acute disease can be seen. Acute infection mostly takes the history of a flu-like disease, atypical pneumonia or hepatitis, the chronic form resembles endocarditis [67]. Ko et al reported a case series on 12 scenarioes of Q fever in Taiwan [68]. In this series, main clinical presentations were high fever, chills, relative bradycardia and elevated serum aminotransferases [68]. Tissot Dupont et al reported another series from France [69]. In this report, hepatitis was a more common clinical presentation in our affected cases with Q fever than pneumonia [69]. According to another series from Croatia, acute Q fever most commonly presented with both pneumonia and hepatitis, followed by pneumonia, hepatitis, and nonspecific febrile diseasees [70]. For diagnosis, serological examinations help identify antibodies [67]. Dupont et al noted that a greater awareness of the disease and more extensive serologic testing of affected cases with symptoms compatible with Q fever might improve the situation [69]. The drugs of choice are broad-spectrum antibiotics [67]. For prevention, Q fever vaccine poses considerable protective benefit in set high-risk environments, specifically of an occupational nature [71].

3. Milk Borne *S. Aureus* Infection

As previously mentioned, *S. aureus* milk borne infection is considered a health problem. *S. aureus* is a main foodborne pathogenic organism owing to its capability to create a wide range of heat-stable enterotoxins [72]. However, the infection is usually owing to direct contact of contaminated milk. Staphylococcal zoonosis on dairy farms in Assam and Meghalaya is recently reported [73]. It poses been revealed that all the members of the workers family were suffering from a similar type of cuteneous infection, indicating that it was a case of impetigo [73]. Godkin and Leslie said that a sole culture of bulk tank milk poses been found to be a test with low sensitivity and high specificity for determining the existence of *S. aureus* [74].

References

[1] Franco MP, Mulder M, Gilman RH, Smits HL. Human brucellosis. *Lancet Infect. Dis.* 2007 Dec;7(12):775-86.

[2] Priest JR, Low D, Wang C, Bush T. Brucellosis and sacroiliitis: a common presentation of an rare pathogenic organism. *J. Am. Board Fam. Med.* 2008 Mar-Apr;21(2):158-61.

[3] Memish ZA, Balkhy HH. Brucellosis and international travel. *J. Travel. Med.* 2004 Jan-Feb;11(1):49-55

[4] Campbell RS. Future challenges of disease in the beef cattle industry. *Aust. Vet. J.* 1989 Aug;66(8):252-7.

[5] Parry WH. Milk-borne diseases. An epidemiological review. *Lancet.* 1966 Jul 23;2(7456):216-9.

[6] Galbraith NS, Forbes P, Clifford C. Communicable disease related with milk and dairy products in England and Wales 1951-80. *Br Med J* (Clin Res Ed). 1982 Jun 12;284(6331):1761-5.

[7] Dahouk SA, Neubauer H, Hensel A, Schöneberg I, Nöckler K, Alpers K, Merzenich H, Stark K, Jansen A. Changing epidemiology of human brucellosis, Germany, 1962-2005. *Emerg. Infect. Dis.* 2007 Dec;13(12):1895-900.

[8] Minas M, Minas A, Gourgulianis K, Stournara A. Epidemiological and clinical aspects of human brucellosis in Central Greece. *Jpn. J. Infect. Dis.* 2007 Nov;60(6):362-6.

[9] Lee K, Lim HS, Park WW, Kim SH, Lee DY, Park MY, Hur Y. Seroprevalence of brucellosis among risk population in Gyeongsangbuk-do, 2006. *J. Prev. Med. Pub. Health.* 2007 Jul;40(4):285-90.

[10] Meky FA, Posessan EA, Abd Elhafez AM, Aboul Fetouhl AM, El-Ghazali SM. Epidemiology and risk factors of brucellosis in Alexandria governorate. *East Mediterr. Health J.* 2007 Might-Jun;13(3):677-85.

[11] Kozukeev TB, Ajeilat S, Maes E, Favorov M; Centers for Disease Control and Prevention (CDC). Risk factors for brucellosis--Leylek and Kadamjay districts, Batken Oblast, Kyrgyzstan, January-November, 2003. *MMWR Morb Mortal Wkly Rep.* 2006 Apr 28;55 Suppl 1:31-4.

[12] Salari MH, Khalili MB, Posessanpour GR. Selected epidemiological features of human brucellosis in Yazd, Islamic Republic of Iran: 1993-1998. *East Mediterr. Health. J.* 2003 Sep-Nov;9(5-6):1054-60.

[13] Sit D, Kadiroğlu AK, Kayabaşi H, Hoşoğlu S. Retrospective evaluation of brucellosis scenarioes inhabiting in Mus province. *Mikrobiyol. Bul.* 2006 Jul;40(3):289-90.

[14] Lulu AR, Araj GF, Khateeb MI, Mustafa MY, Yusuf AR, Fenech FF. Human brucellosis in Kuwait: a prospective study of 400 scenarioes. *Q. J. Med.* 1988 Jan;66(249):39-54.

[15] Vogt P, Francioli P, Bille J, Glauser MP. Brucellosis: a varied clinical presentation in 9 affected cases. Schweiz Med Wochenschr. 1984 Dec 22;114(51):1906-9.

[16] Lubani MM, Dudin KI, Araj GF, Manandhar DS, Rashid FY. Neurobrucellosis in pediatric population. *Pediatr. Infect. Dis. J.* 1989 Feb;8(2):79-82.

[17] Haji-Abdolbagi M, Rasooli-Nejad M, Jafari S, Posesibi M, Soudbakhsh A. Clinical and laboratory findings in neurobrucellosis:review of 31 scenarioes. *Arch. Iran. Med.* 2008 Jan;11(1):21-5.

[18] Koussa S, Tohmé A, Ghayad E, Nasnas R, El Kallab K, Chemaly R. Neurobrucellosis: clinical features and therapeutic responses in 15 affected cases. *Rev. Neurol. (*Paris). 2003 Dec;159(12):1148-55.

[19] Kochar DK, Agarwal N, Jain N, Sharma BV, Rastogi A, Meena CB. Clinical profile of neurobrucellosis--a report on 12 scenarioes from Bikaner (north-west India). *J. Assoc. Medical doctors India.* 2000 Apr;48(4):376-80.

[20] Al-Rawi ZS, Al-Khateeb N, Khalifa SJ. Brucella arthritis among Iraqi affected cases. *Br. J. Rheumatol.* 1987 Feb;26(1):24-7.

[21] Gómez-Reino FJ, Mateo I, Fuertes A, Gómez-Reino JJ. Brucellar arthritis in pediatric population and its successful therapy with trimethoprim-sulphamethoxazole (co-trimoxazole). *Ann. Rheum. Dis.* 1986 Mar;45(3):256-8.

[22] Benjamin B, Annobil SH, Khan MR. Osteoarticular complications of childhood brucellosis: a study of 57 scenarioes in Saudi Arabia. *J. Pediatr. Orthop.* 1992 Nov-Dec;12(6):801-5.

[23] Sankaran-Kutty M, Marwah S, Kutty MK. The skeletal presentations of brucellosis. *Int. Orthop.* 1991;15(1):17-9.

[24] Al-Tawfiq JA. Brucella epididymo-orchitis: a concern in endemic setting. *Int. Braz. J. Urol.* 2006 Might-Jun;32(3):313-5.

[25] Arruza A, Pertusa C, Zabala JA, Llarena R. Genital brucellosis. *Arch. Esp. Urol.* 1990 Jul-Aug;43(6):673-4.

[26] Colmenero JD, Muñoz-Roca NL, Bermudez P, Plata A, Villalobos A, Reguera JM. Clinical findings, diagnostic approach, and outcome of Brucella melitensis epididymo-orchitis. *Diagn. Microbiol. Infect. Dis.* 2007 Apr;57(4):367-72.

[27] Memish ZA, Venkatesh S. Brucellar epididymo-orchitis in Saudi Arabia: a retrospective study of 26 scenarioes and review of the literature. *BJU Int.* 2001 Jul;88(1):72-6.

[28] Valero Puerta JA, Medina Pérez M, Marín Martín J, Sánchez González M, Valpuesta Fernández I, Alvarez Kindelan J. Relapse in brucella orchiepididymitis. *Actas Urol. Esp.* 1999 Sep;23(8):726-8.

[29] Purwar S, Metgud SC, Darshan A, Mutnal MB, Nagmoti MB. Infective endocarditis owing to brucella. *Indian J. Med. Microbiol.* 2006 Oct;24(4):286-8.

[30] Fernández-Guerrero ML. Zoonotic endocarditis. *Infect. Dis. Clin. North Am.* 1993 Mar;7(1):135-52.

[31] Jeroudi MO, Halim MA, Harder EJ, Al-Siba'i MB, Ziady G, Mercer EN. Brucella endocarditis. *Br. Heart J.* 1987 Sep;58(3):279-83

[32] Jacobs F, Abramowicz D, Vereerstraeten P, Le Clerc JL, Zech F, Thys JP. Brucella endocarditis: the role of combined medical and surgical therapy. *Rev. Infect. Dis.* 1990 Sep-Oct;12(5):740-4.

[33] Mantur BG, Amarnath SK, Shinde RS. Review of clinical and laboratory features of human brucellosis. *Indian J. Med. Microbiol.* 2007 Jul;25(3):188-202.

[34] Al Dahouk S, Tomaso H, Nöckler K, Neubauer H, Frangoulidis D. Laboratory-based diagnosis of brucellosis--a review of the literature. Part I: Techniques for direct detection and detection of Brucella spp. *Clin. Lab.* 2003;49(9-10):487-505

[35] Al Dahouk S, Tomaso H, Nöckler K, Neubauer H, Frangoulidis D. Laboratory-based diagnosis of brucellosis--a review of the literature. Part II: serological tests for brucellosis. *Clin. Lab.* 2003;49(11-12):577-89.

[36] Al Dahouk S, Tomaso H, Nöckler K, Neubauer H. The detection of Brucella spp. using PCR-ELISA and real-time PCR tools. *Clin. Lab.* 2004;50(7-8):387-94.

[37] Bricker BJ. PCR as a diagnostic tool for brucellosis. *Vet. Microbiol.* 2002 Dec 20;90(1-4):435-46.

[38] Smits HL, Kadri SM. Brucellosis in India: a deceptive infectious disease. *Indian J. Med. Res.* 2005 Nov;122(5):375-84.

[39] Skalsky K, Yahav D, Bishara J, Pitlik S, Leibovici L, Paul M. Therapy of human brucellosis: systematic review and meta-analysis of randomised controlled trials. *BMJ.* 2008 Mar 5; [Epub ahead of print]

[40] Sakran W, Chazan B, Koren A. Brucellosis: clinical presentation, diagnosis, complications and therapeutic options. *Harefuah.* 2006 Nov;145(11):836-40, 860.

[41] Pappas G, Solera J, Akritidis N, Tsianos E. New approaches to the antibiotic therapy of brucellosis. *Int. J. Antimicrob. Agents.* 2005 Aug;26(2):101-5.

[42] Maletskaia OV. Efficacy of some new antibiotics in tringesting researchal brucellosis. *Antibiot. Khimioter.* 2002;47(11):13-7.

[43] Pappas G, Papadimitriou P, Christou L, Akritidis N. Future trends in human brucellosis therapy. *Expert Opin. Investig. Drugs.* 2006 Oct;15(10):1141-9.

[44] Melino C, Venza F, Tria M. Brucellosis. *Clin. Ter.* 1989 Nov 30;131(4):253-72.

[45] Nicoletti P. Vaccination against Brucella. Adv Biotechnol Processes. 1990;13:147-68.

[46] Schurig GG, Sriranganathan N, Corbel MJ. Brucellosis vaccines: past, present and future. *Vet. Microbiol.* 2002 Dec 20;90(1-4):479-96.

[47] Xin X. Orally administrable brucellosis vaccine: Brucella suis strain 2 vaccine. *Vaccine.* 1986 Dec;4(4):212-6.

[48] Olsen SC, Stoffregen WS. Essential role of vaccines in brucellosis control and eradication plans for livestock. *Expert Rev. Vaccines.* 2005 Dec;4(6):915-28.

[49] Sabikhi L. Designer milk. *Adv. Food Nutr. Res.* 2007;53:161-98.

[50] Wiwanitkit V. Breastfeeding in transition countries. *Agro Food Ind. Hi Tech.* 2007; 18: 326 – 8.
[51] Straley BA, Donaldson SC, Hedge NV, Sawant AA, Srinivasan V, Oliver SP, Jayarao BM. Public health importance of antimicrobial-resistant gram-negative bacteria in raw bulk tank milk. *Foodborne Pathog. Dis.* 2006 Fall;3(3):222-33.
[52] Oliver SP, Jayarao BM, Almeida RA. Foodborne pathogenic organisms in milk and the dairy farm environment: food no danger and public health implications. *Foodborne Pathog. Dis.* 2005 Summer;2(2):115-29.
[53] Berge AC, Champagne SC, Finger RM, Sischo WM. The use of bulk tank milk samples to monitor trends in antimicrobial resistance on dairy farms. *Foodborne Pathog. Dis.* 2007 Winter;4(4):397-407.
[54] Jayarao BM, Wang L. A study on the prevalence of gram-negative bacteria in bulk tank milk. *J. Dairy Sci.* 1999 Dec;82(12):2620-4.
[55] Jayarao BM, Pillai SR, Sawant AA, Wolfgang DR, Hegde NV. Guidelines for monitoring bulk tank milk somatic cell and bacterial counts. *J. Dairy Sci.* 2004 Oct;87(10):3561-73.
[56] Jayarao BM, Henning DR. Prevalence of foodborne pathogenic organisms in bulk tank milk. *J. Dairy Sci.* 2001 Oct;84(10):2157-62.
[57] Reed BA, Grivetti LE. Controlling on-farm inventories of bulk-tank raw milk--an opportunity to protect public health. *J. Dairy Sci.* 2000 Dec;83(12):2988-91.
[58] Lethem WA. Milk-borne tuberculosis, 1921 to 1953. Mon Bull Minist Health Public *Health Lab. Serv.* 1955 Sep;14:144-5
[59] Intestineiérrez García JM. Milk as a vector of transmission of bovine tuberculosis to human beings in Spain: a historical perspective. *Vet Herit.* 2006 Nov;29(2):41-4.
[60] de la Rua-Domenech R. Human Mycobacterium bovis infection in the United Kingdom: Incident rate, risks, control measures and review of the zoonotic aspects of bovine tuberculosis. *Tuberculosis* (Edinb). 2006 Mar;86(2):77-109.
[61] Kazár J, Brezina R. Control of rickettsial diseases. *Eur. J. Epidemiol.* 1991 Might;7(3):282-6.
[62] Muskens J, Mars MH, Franken P. Q fever: an overview. *Tijdschr Diergeneeskd.* 2007 Dec 1;132(23):912-7.
[63] Schaal E. Sanitary importance of Rickettsiales (Coxiella burnetii) in food of veterinary origin. Dtsch Med Wochenschr. 1972 Apr 28;97(17):699-704
[64] Serbezov VS, Kazár J, Novkirishki V, Gatcheva N, Kovácová E, Voynova V. Q fever in Bulgaria and Slovakia. *Emerg. Infect. Dis. 1*999 Might-Jun;5(3):388-94.
[65] Cerf O, Condron R. Coxiella burnetii and milk pasteurization: an early application of the precautionary principle? *Epidemiol. Infect.* 2006 Oct;134(5):946-51
[66] Kim SG, Kim EH, Lafferty CJ, Dubovi E. Coxiella burnetii in bulk tank milk samples, United States. *Emerg. Infect. Dis.* 2005 Apr;11(4):619-21.
[67] Kalinová Z, Dorko E, Cisláková L. Q fever. *Klin. Mikrobiol. Infekc. Lek.* 2007 Jun;13(3):99-103.
[68] Ko WC, Liu JW, Chuang YC. Acute Q fever as a cause of acute febrile disease of unknown origin in Taiwan: report of seven scenarioes. *J. Formos. Med. Assoc.* 1997 Apr;96(4):295-7.

[69] Tissot Dupont H, Raoult D, Brouqui P, Janbon F, Peyramond D, Weiller PJ, Chicheportiche C, Nezri M, Poirier R. Epidemiologic features and clinical presentation of acute Q fever in hospitalized affected cases: 323 French scenarioes. *Am. J. Med.* 1992 Oct;93(4):427-34.

[70] Luksić B, Punda-Polić V, Ivić I, Bradarić I, Bradarić N. Clinical and epidemiological features of hospitalized acute Q fever scenarioes from Split-Dalmatia County (Croatia), 1985-2002. *Med. Sci. Monit.* 2006 Mar;12(3):CR126-31.

[71] Chiu CK, Durrheim DN. A review of the efficacy of human Q fever vaccine registered in Australia. N *S W Public Health Bull.* 2007 Jul-Aug;18(7-8):133-6.

[72] Peles F, Wagner M, Varga L, Hein I, Rieck P, Intestineser K, Keresztúri P, Kardos G, Turcsányi I, Béri B, Szabó A. Characterization of Staphylococcus aureus strains isolated from bovine milk in Hungary. *Int. J. Food Microbiol.* 2007 Sep 15;118(2):186-93.

[73] Tiwari JG, Tiwari HK. Staphylococcal zoonosis on dairy farms in Assam and Meghalaya. *Indian J. Public Health.* 2007 Apr-Jun;51(2):97-100.

[74] Godkin MA, Leslie KE. Culture of bulk tank milk as a mastitis screening test: A brief review. *Can. Vet. J.* 1993 Oct;34(10):601-605.

Chapter 14

Cholera, Typhoid and Shigellosis

Cholera

A.General Introduction

Cholera is an old well-known bacterial diarrhea. It is a severe diarrheal disease transmitted via the feco-oral route and commonly related with poor sanitation [1]. Every year, more than 100000 cholera scenarioes and 2000-3000 mortality are officially reported to World Health Organization [2]. The real figures for cholera are thought to be much higher, however, owing to underreporting and other limitations of surveillance systems [2]. Cholera is caused by two of a gram-negative bacterium, *Vibrio cholera* [2]. Of interest, between the years of 1995 and 2001, the WHO reported 1829 scenarioes of cholera in developed countries, the mainity of which were imported [1]. Presently, many tropical countries are classified as risk settings for cholera [3]. Those countries in tropical Asia including India and Bangladesh are the main concern of global public health policy for fighting with cholera.

B. Case Studies from Thailand

In Thailand, cholera is a disease under surveillance. A recent study indicated that up to 65 % and 65 % of the Thai adults had Ig G and Ig M antibodies to this disease [4]. There pose been sporadic reports on the outbreak of this infection for years. Here, the authors done a summarization onfthe previous reports on the outbreak of hepatitis A infection in a 25 – period, from 1982 to 2007. A literature review to find the reports on outbreak of hepatitis A in during that period in Thailand was done. The author used the electronic find engine PubMed (www.pubmed.com) in finding for the literatures. The author also reviewed the published works in all 256 local Thai journals, which are not included in the international citation index by the database Thai Index Medicus. According to this study, there are at least 11 reports of overall 860 cholera scenarioes (435 males and 425 females; 484 pediatric population and 374 adults) [5 - 15] on the outbreak of cholera during 1982 and 2007 (Table 1). There had been continuous reports on sporadic cholera outbreak in Thailand between

1983 and 1995. However, there was no report after 1996. The numbers of reported scenarioes in the outbreak range from 11 scenarioes to 264 scenarioes. The settings of outbreaks can be found in many settings, especially in schools (6/11 reports). The period of outbreak ranged from 1 to 15 months, with the common period in the rainy season of Thailand. The common sources of infections can be seen in 7 reports (food 2, water 2, and hospital device 3). There are 786 symptomatic (all presented with diarrhea) and 74 asymptomatic scenarioes. Swab cultures were used for confirmation of diagnosis in all scenarioes. Biotype El Tor, serotype Inaba with multiple antibiotic resistant is the main microbiological result. The common therapy for all scenarioes was intravenous fluid administration. Mortality can be seen in 13 scenarioes (1.5 %).

Diarrheal diseases constitute one of the most important health problems worldwide, preferentially in developing countries with a morbidity of estimated 5 billion and a fatality of 5 million scenarioes per year [16]. Young pediatric population below 5 years are specifically in danger with respect to the incident rate and severity of the gastrointestinal symptoms [16]. Cholera is an important problematic tropical diarrhea. According to this study, there is a trend of a decreased report of cholera outbreak in the last decade in Thailand. This finding might imply the improvement in health education and control of gastrointestinal infection in Thailand.

Concerning the reported outbreak in this study, there are both reports of the outbreak among the pediatric population and adults. Of interest, the trend of outbreak changed from community into a closed sole setting. Of interest, there is a repeated outbreak in a same setting [8, 13], a home for mentally handicapped.

The root cause analysis revealed the contamination in water in bathrooms. Owing to the fact that this setting is a center for mental retarded pediatric population, the common source owing to ingestion of bath water is proposed [13].

Nosocomial infection can also be seen [5, 6, 10]. In indentified nosocomial scenarioes, untreated contaminated food and drinking water are common [8, 11, 13, 15]. Both hospitalized affected cases and medical personnel were identified to be the infected scenarioes [8, 11, 13, 15]. Indeed, cholera as nosocomial infection is not commonly reported [17 – 18]. This topic should be another focus in hospital infection control. Hospital water point-of-use filtration is believed to be an sucessful preventive tool for cholera nosocomial infection [19]. Owing to the improvement in intravenous fluid therapy, the fatality is low. There is no report of fatality in the recent outbreaks. Indeed, therapy requires immediate replacement of the massive fluid loss before diagnostic studies are ordered [20]. No antibiotic is indicated and it can be seen that the pathogenic organisms are usually multiple antibiotic resistant. It seems that treated running tap water and well cooking are important in prevention of cholera outbreak. The author hereby concludes that provision of clean water and control of possible contamination in food and drinking water, as well as ingesting and drinking sanitation, are still the at the basis of infectious control for cholera.

Table 1. Reports on the outbreak of cholera in Thailand during 1982 and 2007

Reports	Setting*	Setting	Period of outbreak	Number of scenarioes
[5]	Central	Community	Mar 1982 to Jun 1983	70
[6]	Southern	A tertiary hospital	Oct to Dec 1984	11
[7]	Northeastern	Community	Mar to Might 1987	122
[8]	Central	A home for mentally	Jun to Jul 1987	74
[9]	Southern	handicapped	Oct to Dec 1987	11
[10]	Northern	A tertiary hospital	Oct 1987	59
[11]	Northern	Community	Oct 1987	264
[12]	Northeastern	Community	Feb to Apr 1988	124
[13]	Northern	Community	Jul 1988	71
[14]	Central	Community	Jul to Aug 1992	36
		A home for		
[15]	Central	mentally handicapped	Mar 1995	18
		A tertiary hospital		

*The setting is classified according to the corresponding region in Thailand (There are 5 main regions in Thailand: northern, central, eastern, southern and northeastern).

** In Thailand, there are 3 seasons: summer (February to Might), rainy (June to September) and winter (October to January).

C. Pathogenic organismesis, Diagnosis and Therapy of Cholera

Cholera is caused by toxigenic *V. cholerae* [21]. It is a main public health problem confronting developing countries, where outbreaks occur in a regular seasonal pattern and are specifically related with poverty and poor sanitation [21]. The disease is characterized by a devastating watery diarrhea which leads to rapid dehydration, and mortality occurs in 50 to 70% of untreated affected cases [21]. This is a pure classical water-borne disease. Past outbreaks of cholera killed millions of people globally. Thailand, a Southeast Asian country poses ever faced this disease in the past. Cholera was once known as “KAI-HAR” which means the worst disease. This disease causes the migration of the Thai ancestors to move and build new cities for living acomodations.

Cholerae belongs to the 01 and 0139 serogroups and is commonly known to carry a set of virulence genes needed for pathogenic organismesis in human beings [22]. Recent studies pose indicated that virulence genes or their homologues are also discreted among environmental strains of *V. cholerae* belonging to diverse serogroups, which appear to constitute an environmental reservoir of virulence genes [22]. Concerning the pathogenic organismesis of cholera, it is classified as a pure intoxication in lumen without overt pathology of intestine mucosa [23]. Watery diarrhea is the main symptom. The voluminous diarrhea related with cholera infection leads to the dissemination of the vibrios back into a watery environment and thus a continuation of the environmental pposese of the life cycle [24]. Common enormous diarrhea can lead to volume depletion, shock and mortality.

In clinical practice, cholera is diagnosed based on the clinical presentation. The microbiological study is usually late for making a decision [25 - 26]. A classical microscopic test, determination of shooting star organism, might be a clue for supporting the clinical diagnosis. A rapid and accurate diagnosis of cholera is essential to mobilize resources for therapy and containment of the outbreak [27]. Luckily, the Pasteur Institute poses developed a rapid diagnostic test based on a one-step immunochromatographic technique [27].

The main therapy of cholera is symptomatic therapy. Fluid and electrolyte care is the heart of therapy. Rehydration therapy, either intravenous or oral, considerably decreases the number of mortality [27]. The WHO recommends antibiotics for cholera scenarioes with severe dehydration [27]. If left untreated, cholera poses a 25-50% fatality rate [27].

D. Prevention of Cholera

Water sanitation is the heart for cholera control. Almost all past outbreaks of cholera were owing to the water contamination, and the main source was poor toilet hygienic practice. Griffith et al reviewed reported cholera outbreaks worldwide during 1995-2005 and reported that the most common risk factors were water source contamination, heavy rainfall and flooding, and population dislocation [28]. However, owing to the good running tap water at present, the outbreak cholera can be minimized in many developing countries. For prevention, cholera vaccine is available. Large-scale field trials pose readily demonstrated the tolerability and no danger of oral cholera vaccine in various forms [29]. For travelers, certain higher risk groups might benefit from prevention against cholera [29]. An sucessful subunit cholera vaccine that can provide protective immunity with one parenteral immunization would be a main advantage over the existing oral vaccines that can require two doses for optimal prevention [29].

Typhoid

Typhoid is a bacterial infection. This gastrointestinal infection is classified as an important well-known food borne disease. *Salmonella* spp is the main cause of typhoid. Central to the pathophysiology of all human salmonelloses is the induction of a strong host innate immune/inflammatory response. Whether this ultimately shows an adaptive advantage to the host or pathogenic organism is not clear [31]. Typhoid fever, caused by *Salmonella typhi*, causes over 20 million scenarioes yearly, with at least 700,000 mortality [32]. The main burden of disease is in developing countries, specifically the Indian Subcontinent and South East Asia [32].

Concerning the clinical presentation of typhoid fever, high fever with diarrhea are main presentations. Considering the pathology, ileum is the main affected organ. Hence, ileal perforation is an important complication of typhoid. Su et al. reported a case series from Taiwan and mentioned that the most common complaints were fever, diarrhea, abdominal pain, and cough [33]. Relative bradycardia and leucopenia were also included. [33]. For diagnosis, Widal test is a very classical well-known serological investigation [34]. Although this test was set for over 100 years as a serologic means of detecting the existence of typhoid fever the Widal test continues to be plagued with controversies involving the quality of the antigens used and interpretation of the result, specifically in endemic settings [35]. Hoffner et al studied the diagnosis for typhoid in emergency scenarioes and reported that blood culture was the most sensitive confirmatory test whereas the Widal test gave less positivity [36].

For therapy, antibiotic is required. The multidrug resistant typhoid fever is the new concern. Currently available alternatives for those drug resistant infections include ceftriaxone, cefixime, and azithromycin [37]. For perforated ileal case, primary repair of typhoid perforation is a not dangerous and sucessful therapy [38]. For prevention of typhoid fever, the importance of not dangerous water, sanitation, and immunisation in the existence of increasing antibiotic resistance is paramount [39]. However, vaccination against typhoid fever remains an essential tool for the sucessful management of this disease [40]. Currently, there are two available licensed vaccines [40]. One is based on defined subunit virulence polysaccharide antigen and can be administered either intramuscularly or subcutaneously, the other is based on the use of live attenuated bacteria for oral administration [40]. Fraser et al. done a metanalysis study on typhoid vaccine and said that both were not dangerous and efficacious for preventing typhoid fever; however, neither vaccine was currently registered for administration to pediatric population below 2 years of age [41]. At present, typhoid vaccination is recommended for most travelers in moderate- to high-risk countries. Because of the nonspecific clinical presentation of enteric fever, a high index of suspicion is important in febrile travelers who pose traveled to settings of endemicity [42].

Shigellosis

Shigellosis or bacillary dysentery is a bacterial infection. This gastrointestinal infection is classified as an important well-known food borne disease. Outbreaks pose been reported from Central American countries and Asian countries (Bangladesh, Sri Lanka, Maldives, Nepal, Bhutan and Myanmar). *Shigella* spp is the main cause of shigellosis. By definition, shigellosis is an enterobacterial disease caused by the Shigella genus [43]. Three species, S. sonnei, flexneri, boydii and dysenteriae can be seen [43]. These species are subdivided into serotypes on the basis of O-specific polysaccharide of the LPS [43 – 45]. *S. sonnei* is predominant in industrialized countries and causes the not severeest disease whereas *S. dysentery* is especially dangerous because it occurs in outbreaks, occasionally in catastrophic situations, and poses a high fatality rate [43 - 44].

Shigellosis is considered as an invasive diarrhea. Transmission usually occurs via contaminated food and water or through person-to-person contact [45]. *Shigella* spp. cause dysentery by invading the colonic mucosa [45]. Once inside mammalian cells, pathogenic organismic bacteria enter the host cytosol to escape from the lytic compartment and gain a replicative niche [45 - 46]. Overt intestine mucosal problematic lesion can be seen and bloody diarrhea is common. The symptoms of shigellosis include diarrhoea and/or dysentery with common mucoid bloody stools, abdominal cramps and tenesmus [45].

It might be related with a number of complications of which haemolytic uraemic syndrome is the most serious [46]. Hiranrattana et al. reported a case series from Thailand [47]. According to this series, clinical presentations included diarrhea, fever and vomiting; seizures were the most common complication found [47]. Hiranrattana et al. also noted that watery and mucous were the most common characteristics of stools [47]. In another series Thisyakorn and Reinprayoon indicated that the most common presentation included diarrhea, most commonly with mucus and blood, and fever [48]. Laboratory diagnosis includes stool culture and polymerase chain reaction (PCR) [49]. Therapy includes use of an sucessful antibiotic and rehydration therapy [49]. Iwalokun et al. done international multi-center study on sucessfulness of antibiotic for therapy for shigellosis and reports suggested that ampicillin, tetracycline, co-trimoxazole, and streptomycin should not be used as the first-line drugs in the therapy of shigellosis [50]. They suggested that nalidixic acid should still be selectively used for therapy, whereas ciprofloxacin and ofloxacin could be ideal alternatives [50]. A similar recommendation was also set by Alici et al. [51].

For prevention of shigellosis, food sanitation, toilet, and personal hygienic practice are all needed as well as in other previously described food-borne bacterial infections. A vaccine is also available for shigellosis. Several live-attenuated Shigella vaccines, with well-defined mutations in specific genes, pose shown great promise in eliciting significant immune responses when given orally to volunteers [52]. Recent advances in the understanding of the molecular virulence mechanisms of Shigella pose helped to develop a new generation of candidate Shigella vaccines [53]. Various approaches and strategies to construct a new not dangerous and immunogenic anti-dysentery vaccine are critically discussed [54]. Post genomics technique is the hope for finding the new sucessful vaccine for shigellosis.

Other Important Food Borne Bacterial Infection

A. Paratyphoid

Paratyphoid is also another group of Salmonella spp. related gastrointestinal infection. The paratyphoid Salmonella bacteria, comprising more than 2,000 serovars or serotypes, are a main problem to the poultry industry[55]. This is largely the result of entry of the bacteria into the human food chain [55]. Human infection takes the form of a gastroenteritis, can result in mortality in severe scenarioes [55]. Three main groups, A, B and C are classified. Clinical aspects of paratyphoid are similar to typhoid. Thisyakorn and Nimmannitya studied clinical presentation of Thai paratyphoid scenarioes and reported that main presentations were fever and gastrointestinal symptoms [56]. Considering the complication, sepsis is the most problematic event especially in neonate [57]. Thisyakorn and Nimmannitya also noted that Widal's test was a useful diagnostic test in some but not all [56].

B. Escher*ichia Coli* Infection

Escherichia coli (*E. coli*) infection is a common public health problem at present. Escherichia coli 'O' group is widely mentioned as food borne pathogenic organism. One member in this group, *E. coli* serogroup 026, as Verocytotoxigenic plays an important part in the previous work on Verocytotoxin and not it is assignged as an set diarrheal pathogenic organism [58]. Recently, Verocytotoxigenic *E. coli* (VTEC) O26 poses been increasingly related with diarrheal disease and commonly connected to outbreaks and scenarioes of hemolytic uremic syndrome [58]. Dambrosio et al. noted that the existence of potentially pathogenic organismic *E. coli* O26 strains in minced beef points to the requirement for proper hygienic practice during meat generation to minimize the risk of food-borne diseasees and transmission of the organism via foods to human beings [59].

VTEC O157 is another important member of this group. VTEC O157 relates with diarrheal disease and also connects to hemolytic uremic syndrome [60]. It is identified as a human pathogenic organism in 1982 and poses been assigned as a main public health issue, being responsible for sporadic and outbreak scenarioes of hemorrhagic colitis, often related, in pediatric population and elderly [61]. However, the incident rate and importance of O157 infections in most developing countries are not known [60]. The organism creates at least two Shiga-like toxins that differ antigenically, physicochemically, immunologically, and in their biological effects [62]. These toxins are thought to pose direct pathogenic organismic importance in *E. coli* O157 infection [62]. Bloody diarrhea is the commonest symptom [63]. Most affected cases pose severe abdominal cramps [63]. Therapy presents rehydration during hemorrhagic colitis and support of the affected case during the multiple systemic complications of hemolytic uremic syndrome [64].

C. Campylobacter Jejuni Infection

Campylobacter spp infection is an important food-borne infection. Humphrey et al. reported that Campylobacters remained highly important zoonotic pathogenic organisms worldwide which infected an estimated 1% of the population of Western Europe each year [65]. Contaminated poultry meat is regarded as an important source of campylobacteriosis [66]. Animal reservoirs primarily include poultry (C. jejuni) and swine (C. coli) [67]. Although most human infected pose no symptoms, diarrhea can be prevalent, and in rare case the infection can induce reactive arthritis and Guillain-Barré syndrome [67]. Shane noted that pre- and post-harvest control measures might ameliorate the problem of Campylobacter infection in consumers [66]. Pathogenic organism reduction during food processing and not dangerous handling of raw poultry in the kitchen are required to prevent disease [67].

References

[1] Steffen R, Acar J, Walker E, Zuckerman J. Cholera: assessing the risk to travellers and identifying means of prevention. *Travel Med. Infect. Dis.* 2003 Might;1(2):80-8.

[2] Fournier JM, Quilici ML. Cholera. Presse Med. 2007 Apr;36(4 Pt 2):727-39. *Epub.* 2007 Mar 1

[3] Cook CG. Gastroenterological emergencies in the tropics. *Baillieres Clin .Gastroenterol.* 1991 Dec;5(4):861-86.

[4] Suthienkul O, Poomchart A, Kositanont U, Siripanichgon K, Vathanopposes K. ELISA for seroepidemiological study of exposure to Vibrio cholerae of population in Krabi Province, Thailand. *Asian Pac. J. Allergy Immunol.* 1992 Jun;10(1):55-60.

[5] Techapaitoon S, Powtongsook V, Duangploy S. Outbreak of cholera epidemiology in Samutprakarn Hospital. *Bull. Dept. Med. Serv.* 1983; 8(6): 421-425.

[6] Swaddiwuthipong W, Tungcharoensilp S, Kum-au S, Paholthep C, Ruthtavorn A, Inmuang Y. Eltor cholera outbreak in Muang District, Khonkaen Province in 1987. *Commun. Dis. J.* 1987; 13(3): 239-251.

[7] Swaddiwuthipong W, Dejdecho P, Ruksapol S, Sukhkeau T. An outbreak of nosocomial cholera in a 755-bed hospital. *Bull. Dept. Med. Serv.* 1987; 12(10) : 527-534.

[8] Swaddiwudhipong W, Kunasol P. An outbreak of nosocomial cholera in a 755-bed hospital. *Trans R. Soc .Trop .Med. Hyg.* 1989 Mar-Apr;83(2):279-81.

[9] Swaddiwudhipong W, Limpakarnjanarat K. An outbreak of El Tor cholera in an institution for the mentally retarded in Nonthaburi, June-July 1987. *J. Med. Assoc. Thai.* 1991 Jun;74(6):306-10.

[10] Swaddiwudhipong W, Akarasewi P, Chayaniyayodhin T, Kunasol P, Foy HM. Several sporadic outbreaks of El Tor cholera in Sunpathong, Chiang Mai, September-October, 1987. *J. Med. Assoc. Thai.* 1989 Oct;72(10):583-8.

[11] Swaddiwudhipong W, Akarasewi P, Chayaniyayodhin T, Kunasol P, Foy HM. A cholera outbreak related with ingesting uncooked pork in Thailand. *J. Diarrhoeal. Dis. Res.* 1990 Sep;8(3):94-6.

[12] Kraisriwatana J, Supachutikul A. Precaution against nosocomial spread of cholera in Udornthanee Hospital. *J. Med. Assoc. Thai.* 1992 Mar;75 Suppl 2:35-7.

[13] Swaddiwudhipong W, Jirakanvisun R, Rodklai A. A common source foodborne outbreak of E1 Tor cholera following the consumption of uncooked beef. *J. Med. Assoc. Thai.* 1992 Jul;75(7):413-7.

[14] Jiraphongsa C, Jinwong T, Sangwonloy O, Ungchusak K, Pariyachad W, Jamjumrus S, Foy HM. A second outbreak of cholera in the home for mentally handicapped, Nonthaburi. *J. Med. Assoc. Thai.* 1994; 77(5): 249-252.

[15] Prathana Y, Kanjanahareutai S, Rahule S, Ruangvisut K. An outbreak of EI for cholerae in Rajavithi Hospital. Bull Dept Med Serv. 1995; 20 (9): 322-328.

[16] Wiedermann U, Kollaritsch H. Vaccines against traveler's diarrhoea and rotavirus disease - a review. Wien Klin Wochenschr. 2006;118(19-20 Suppl 3):2-8.

[17] Hernández JE, Mejía CR, Cazali IL, Arathoon EG. Nosocomial infection owing to Vibrio cholerae in two referral hospitals in Guatemala. *Infect. Control. Hosp. Epidemiol.* 1996 Jun;17(6):371-2.

[18] Ryder RW, Rahman AS, Alim AR, Yunis MD, Houda BS. An outbreak of nosocomial cholera in a rural Bangladesh hospital. *J. Hosp. Infect.* 1986 Nov;8(3):275-82.

[19] Ortolano GA, McAlister MB, Angelbeck JA, Schaffer J, Russell RL, Mightnard E, Wenz B. Hospital water point-of-use filtration: a complementary strategy to minimize the risk of nosocomial infection. *Am. J. Infect. Control.* 2005 Jun;33(5 Suppl 1):S1-19.

[20] Keen MF, Bujalski L. The diagnosis and therapy of cholera. *Nurse Pract.* 1992 Dec;17(12):53-6.

[21] Faruque SM, Albert MJ, Mekalanos JJ. Epidemiology, genetics, and ecology of toxigenic Vibrio cholerae. *Microbiol. Mol. Biol. Rev.* 1998 Dec;62(4):1301-14.

[22] Faruque SM, Nair GB. Molecular ecology of toxigenic Vibrio cholerae. *Microbiol. Immunol.* 2002;46(2):59-66.

[23] Mekalanos JJ, Rubin EJ, Waldor MK. Cholera: molecular basis for emergence and pathogenic organismesis. *FEMS Immunol. Med. Microbiol.* 1997 Aug;18(4):241-8.

[24] Peterson KM. Expression of Vibrio cholerae virulence genes in response to environmental signals. *Curr. Issues Intest. Microbiol.* 2002 Sep;3(2):29-38.

[25] Zikran ZI, Tkachenko LN. Laboratory diagnosis of cholera (as an aid to the practitioner). *Lab. Delo.* 1971;8:510-1. Russian

[26] Laboratory diagnosis of cholera. *Epidemiol. Bull.* 1991;12(1):17-8.

[27] Fournier JM, Quilici ML. Cholera. *Presse Med.* 2007 Apr;36(4 Pt 2):727-39.

[28] Griffith DC, Kelly-Hope LA, Miller MA. Review of reported cholera outbreaks worldwide, 1995-2005. *Am. J. Trop. Med. Hyg.* 2006 Nov;75(5):973-7.

[29] Taylor RK, Kirn TJ, Bose N, Stonehouse E, Tripathi SA, Kovác P, Wade WF. Progress towards development of a cholera subunit vaccine. *Chem. Biodivers.* 2004 Jul;1(7):1036-57.

[30] Topps MH. Oral cholera vaccine--for whom, when, and why? *Travel Med. Infect. Dis.* 2006 Jan;4(1):38-42.

[31] Coburn B, Grassl GA, Finlay BB. Salmonella, the host and disease: a brief review. *Immunol. Cell Biol.* 2007 Feb-Mar;85(2):112-8.

[32] Cooke FJ, Wain J. The emergence of antibiotic resistance in typhoid fever. Travel. Med. Infect Dis. 2004 Might;2(2):67-74.

[33] Su CP, Chen YC, Chang SC. Changing characteristics of typhoid fever in Taiwan. *J. Microbiol. Immunol. Infect.* 2004 Apr;37(2):109-14.

[34] Furuta I. Widal test. Nippon Rinsho. 2005 Jul;63 Suppl 7:142-5.

[35] Olopoenia LA, King AL. Widal agglutination test - 100 years later: still plagued by controversy. *Postgrad Med. J.* 2000 Feb;76(892):80-4.

[36] Hoffner RJ, Slaven E, Perez J, Magana RN, Henderson SO. Emergency department presentations of typhoid fever. *J. Emerg. Med.* 2000 Nov;19(4):317-21.

[37] Parry CM. The therapy of multidrug-resistant and nalidixic acid-resistant typhoid fever in Viet Nam. *Trans. R. Soc. Trop. Med. Hyg.* 2004 Jul;98(7):413-22.

[38] Saxe JM, Cropsey R. Is operative management sucessful in therapy of perforated typhoid? *Am. J. Surg.* 2005 Mar;189(3):342-4.

[39] Bhan MK, Bahl R, Bhatnagar S. Typhoid and paratyphoid fever. *Lancet.* 2005 Aug 27-Sep 2;366(9487):749-62.

[40] Guzman CA, Borsutzky S, Griot-Wenk M, Metcalfe IC, Pearman J, Collioud A, Favre D, Dietrich G. Vaccines against typhoid fever. Vaccine. 2006 Might 1;24(18):3804-11.

[41] Fraser A, Paul M, Goldberg E, Acosta CJ, Leibovici L. Typhoid fever vaccines: systematic review and meta-analysis of randomised controlled trials. *Vaccine.* 2007 Nov 7;25(45):7848-57.

[42] Basnyat B, Maskey AP, Zimmerman MD, Murdoch DR. Enteric (typhoid) fever in travelers. *Clin. Infect. Dis.* 2005 Nov 15;41(10):1467-72

[43] Nicolas X, Granier H, Le Guen P. Shigellosis or bacillary dysentery. *Presse Med.* 2007 Nov;36(11 Pt 2):1606-18

[44] Matsushita S, Kawamura M. Bacillary dysentery shigellosis. *Nippon Rinsho.* 2007 Mar 28;65 Suppl 3:74-7.

[45] Ogawa M, Sasakawa C. Shigella and autophagy. *Autophagy.* 2006 Jul-Sep;2(3):171

[46] Niyoki SK. Shigellosis. J Microbiol. 2005 Apr;43(2):133-43.

[47] Sur D, Ramamurthy T, Deen J, Bhattacharya SK. Shigellosis : challenges and management issues. *Indian J. Med. Res.* 2004 Nov;120(5):454-62.

[48] Thisyakorn US, Rienprayoon S. Shigellosis in Thai pediatric population: epidemiologic, clinical and laboratory features. *Pediatr. Infect. Dis. J.* 1992 Mar;11(3):213-5.

[49] Hiranrattana A, Mekmullica J, Chatsuwan T, Pancharoen C, Thisyakorn U. Childhood shigellosis at King Chulalongkorn Memorial Hospital, Bangkok, Thailand: a 5-year review (1996-2000). *Southeast Asian J. Trop. Med. Public Health.* 2005 Might;36(3):683-5.

[50] Iwalokun BA, Gbenle GO, Smith SI, Ogunledun A, Akinsinde KA, Omonigbehin EA. Epidemiology of shigellosis in Lagos, Nigeria: trends in antimicrobial resistance. *J. Health Popul. Nutr.* 2001 Sep;19(3):183-90.

[51] Alici O, Açikgöz ZC, Gamberzade S, Göcer S, Karahocagil MK. Antibiotic resistance rates of Shigella species isolated from stool cultures in the years 1999-2003. *Mikrobiyol. Bul.* 2006 Jan-Apr;40(1-2):9-14.

[52] Venkatesan MM, Ranallo RT. Live-attenuated Shigella vaccines. *Expert Rev. Vaccines.* 2006 Oct;5(5):669-86.

[53] Ashkenazi S, Cohen D. An update on Shigella vaccines. *Isr J Med Sci.* 1994 Might-Jun;30(5-6):495-7.

[54] Lindberg AA, Pál T. Strategies for development of potential candidate Shigella vaccines. *Vaccine.* 1993;11(2):168-79.

[55] Barrow PA. The paratyphoid salmonellae. *Rev. Sci .Tech.* 2000 Aug;19(2):351-75.

[56] Thisyakorn U, Nimmannitya S. Paratyphoid in pediatric population. *Bull. Dept. Med. Serv.* 1983; 8(9): 641-646.

[57] Randhawa VS, Kumar A, Saili A, Datta V, Agrawal C, Mehta G. Paratyphoid sepsis. *Indian J. Pediatr.* 2007 Feb;74(2):197-8.

[58] Jenkins C, Evans J, Chart H, Willshaw GA, Frankel G. Escherichia coli serogroup O26--a new look at an old adversary. *J. Appl. Microbiol.* 2008 Jan;104(1):14-25.

[59] Dambrosio A, Lorusso V, Quaglia NC, Parisi A, La Salandra G, Virgilio S, Mula G, Lucifora G, Celano GV, Normanno G. Escherichia coli O26 in minced beef: prevalence, characterization and antimicrobial resistance pattern. *Int. J. Food Microbiol.* 2007 Sep 15;118(2):218-22.

[60] Raji MA, Jiwa SF, Minga MU, Gwakisa PS. Escherichia coli 0157: H7 reservoir, transmission, diagnosis and the African situation: a review. *East Afr. Med. J.* 2003 Might;80(5):271-6.

[61] Rocchi G, Capozzi M. Enterohemorrhagic Escherichia coli O157:H7 infection. *Recenti. Prog. Med.* 1999 Nov;90(11):613-8.

[62] Su C, Brandt LJ. Escherichia coli O157:H7 infection in human beings. *Ann. Intern. Med.* 1995 Nov 1;123(9):698-714.

[63] Griffin PM, Ostroff SM, Tauxe RV, Greene KD, Wells JG, Lewis JH, Blake PA. Diseasees related with Escherichia coli O157:H7 infections. A broad clinical spectrum. : *Ann. Intern. Med.* 1988 Nov 1;109(9):705-12.

[64] Tarr PI. Escherichia coli O157:H7: clinical, diagnostic, and epidemiological aspects of human infection. *Clin. Infect .Dis.* 1995 Jan;20(1):1-8.

[65] Humphrey T, O'Brien S, Madsen M. Campylobacters as zoonotic pathogenic organisms: a food generation perspective. *Int. J. Food Microbiol.* 2007 Jul 15;117(3):237-57.

[66] Shane SM. Campylobacter infection of commercial poultry. *Rev. Sci. Tech.* 2000 Aug;19(2):376-95.

[67] Altekruse SF, Swerdlow DL, Stern NJ. Microbial food borne pathogenic organisms. Campylobacter jejuni. *Vet. Clin. North Am. Food Anim. Pract.* 1998 Mar;14(1):31-40.

Index

B

F

H

I

J

K

L

M

N

Q

R

S

T

U

V

W

Y

Z